Aromatherapy Secrets for Wellness

Maximize Your Life Force, Transform Stress and Conquer Ailments with Essential Oils

by

Marina Dufort, R.A.

(Marina Mermaid)

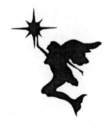

Aromatherapy Secrets for Wellness:
Maximize Your Life Force, Transform Stress and Conquer Ailments
with Essential Oils

ISBN 10: 0-9848462-1-2
ISBN 13: 978-0-9848462-1-4

Published by Expert Author Publishing
http://expertauthorpublishing.com

Canadian Address

1265 Charter Hill Drive
Coquitlam, BC, V3E 1P1
Phone: (604) 941-3041
Fax: (604) 944-7993

US Address

1300 Boblett Street
Unit A-218
Blaine, WA 98230
Phone: (866) 492-6623
Fax: (250) 493-6603

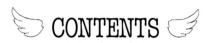 CONTENTS

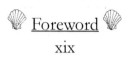

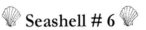

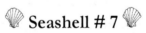 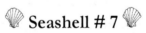
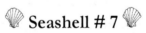 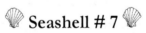
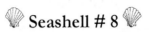
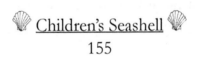 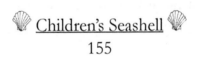
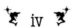

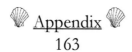

Praise for Aromatherapy Secrets for Wellness

How Marina and the Oils Helped Fight Cancer . . .

I was diagnosed with stage three colon cancer that spread into the lymph nodes. My numerous doctors all suggested that I start a vigorous treatment of various chemotherapies right after the tumor was removed. It seemed like everyone was addressing the symptoms and not interested in anything beyond a five-year survival rate. It was then that I started looking into alternative therapies, naturopathic medicine and healing.

I met Marina to discuss olfactory treatments—AKA, aromatherapy—and to begin some reflexology sessions. Being in the care of Marina with all her wisdom and energy is a healing experience of its own. I truly believe that she is gifted, and integrating Western therapies with natural medicine is the future of managing cancer. Not only has my life changed for the better, I know that I am in charge of my path to wellness. Thank you Marina!

Bonnie Barton
Vancouver, B.C.

How Marina and the Oils Relieved My Stress . . .

When I met Marina ten years ago, I was grieving my father's death and I was looking for comfort at a spiritual level. Thanks

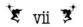

to my beloved son, Anthony, I received an aromatherapy massage from Marina and I felt the shift right away.

The use of essential oils and my connection with Marina started to make me more aware of my energy levels. For me it was a discovery. Finally I started to feel more relaxed and able to receive, after all these years of stress and intense focus building my life in France with my very successful cosmetics business.

I have been using essential oils and holistic services on a regular basis now. I will turn 59 in three months and I am feeling more healthy and vibrant than ever.

Thank you Marina, without you and the aromatherapy massages my life would be different.

Marie-Jeanne Godard, Canada

"What a blissful journey I was able to experience by being placed in the caring hands of Marina! Being a brand new mom can be stressful. **Pump the Peace** spritzer was part of this amazing journey where I was able to calm down from the sound of her caring voice, to the joyful wisdom felt through her hands, to the delicious array of rich smells… It was a Utopian experience!

Being a new mom I have been delightfully devoted to giving for my angel, so it was an experience I needed to receive and give to myself. From this hour on a bed of relaxation and surrender, I was full of bliss and to be able to give more as a mom and to feel whole again. I felt amazing! Marina even brought my baby son Christian, 8 months old, in the room afterward to sit on the bed and absorb the essences in the air and inhale to raw essence of his momma that she drew through her massage… He was in peace, and loved that she took the time to chime (Native Indian chime sound therapy).

Happy momma, happy baby. We both reaped many benefits from our experience on the table at MAA YOGA studio in the hands of a woman who truly has an amazing gift. A gift to heal, rejuvenate, and bring inner peace! One should be honored to experience what Marina offers.

Brei Souza, new mom and staff at
MAA YOGA studio, Deep Cove, B.C., Canada

As a cinematographer on countless TV series and motion pictures for nearly 30 years I have always tried to surround myself with people who are the best at what they do. Marina is one of those people.

Far from being glamorous, work on a film set is usually grueling. With long, long hour days and nights, often in bad weather and miserable locations, the crew was always happier when Marina was there. Her main job as a "stand in" was to repeat the actions of the actors (Including Brooke Shields, Carol Burnett and even Eric Stoltz) so we could set up and light the shots in a way that made actors look like the stars they were. That she did this perfectly was important, but more significantly, the light and positive energy she brought every day without fail always lifted everyone's spirits. And if that wasn't enough, she further energized an exhausted crew with her shoulder massages and her own marvelous essential oils and aromatherapy, and even her musical voice.

We all miss her and we all know her book will be excellent. It is the only way she does things!

Robert McLachlan ASC, CSC
Vancouver/ Los Angeles

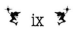

ix

How Marina and the Oils Relieved My Pain . . .

Following a bad car accident, while still in the midst of recovery from a torn gluteus medial muscle, I was left with almost no hope of being able to get back to normal life, work and sports. However, after intensive treatment by Marina, her wonderful blends of essential oils and her magical gift of healing, I can honestly say I am able to run, stretch and I am the most flexible I have been in years despite being 51 years old. Marina worked tirelessly on me initially with mud and seaweed wraps and then the magical blends of oils with her incredible healing hands.

Marina is truly a rare gift to the healing profession and I would recommend her to anyone. Thank you "Marina Mermaid." You truly are a healing Angel.

Andrew M. Bramley, Ph.D.
Pharmacology, London University (UK)
Vancouver, B.C.

I'm not exactly sure how I got to be 53 years old. It seems like I was 30 a few months ago. But, here I am, and, like most men my age, I tend to push my body like I'm still 18. Playing hockey, riding my bike, working out at the gym, it all takes its toll. Every week there's yet another bruise, pulled muscle or aching joint. And now that I'm older they seem to take forever to heal—if they ever do. Recently, my left arm was in particularly bad shape. I couldn't lift it higher than my shoulder without significant pain. Over time it was getting worse, not better. I had to give up riding my bike and pretty much everything else. I didn't know what to do other than just suffer through it for an unknown period of time.

x

Then I went to Marina and she worked her magic. I say "magic" because that's the best word I can use to describe it. She has truly harnessed the power of the natural world and all its healing power. From the moment I walk into her treatment room, I feel I'm in good hands. She understands the human body and the stresses we heap upon it. When she begins her therapy, I feel more relaxed, centered and balanced. The pain just slips away. For my arm specifically, she applied something very special of her own creation; the amazing 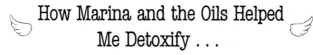 **Mr. Fix It**. Wow, I could feel it working within seconds. I'm not sure exactly what's in it, but I can't say enough about how effective it is. Trust me, it works. I took a small bottle home with clear instructions on how to apply it myself. Thanks to Marina, I'm feeling like I'm 30 years old again. Time to get bike riding!

Thanks Marina!

Scot McDonald, director, producer, videographer
FULL FRAME Productions

How Marina and the Oils Helped Me Detoxify . . .

Now I know why her nickname is Marina Mermaid. But from now on, I will call her "Alchemist Marina Mermaid."

In my 20 years in the fitness industry as a Personal Trainer and a Natural Bodybuilder, I never thought to go for an "aromatherapy" massage. OK, don't tell this to anyone, but I did try it and let me tell you something… WOW! Marina is the top of the line in her field. This is nothing like a regular massage. It's a journey for your senses and a great sensation for your whole body.

As a cancer survivor, I know how important it is to take

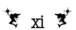

care of your health and the importance of detoxifying the body. I was impressed with Marina's knowledge about all the different sorts of oils. Each essential oil has its own benefit, and Marina, like an alchemist, makes different blends for your specific needs.

Thank you Marina, and you can add my name to your list of regular clients.

Martin Bolduc, CPT, ACE, BCRPA
Author of *The Ultimate Guide to Express Fat Loss*

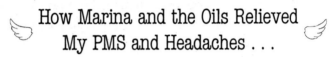

How Marina and the Oils Relieved My PMS and Headaches . . .

Dear Marina,

I wanted to write you a sincere letter of gratitude. Before I met you I had menstrual flow that was so sporadic and heavy at times that it was alarming. I took your advice and rubbed your **Dragon Lady Flush** remedy on my belly followed by a hot compress. I did this just a day prior to my expected period. The results were staggering! My flow was normal and I felt no extreme moments of heavy flow.

I also suffered from pre-menstrual headaches the day before my cycle every month. These headaches could not be relieved by any painkiller. You created a spritzer for me called *Headache Gooone*, which actually eliminated my headache!

I also wanted you to know that the **Pump the Peace** and **Pump the Joy** spritzers that you created are amazing. I keep them at my side and pump a small amount to lift my spirits when needed.

I would recommend your natural therapies to anyone I know. I thank you from the bottom of my heart.

Kindest regards,
Monique Rook
Vancouver, B.C.

How Marina and the Oils Revived My Immunity and Eliminated Colds and Flu . . .

In the two years that I have been having aromatherapy massage sessions with Marina, I have experienced a renewed sense of health and wellbeing, energy and increased immunity from the flu, coughs and colds. As a lawyer I work long hours. The office environment with indoor heating in the winter and air conditioning in the summer means that one person gets sick and then many others also get sick. Since having treatments with Marina, I seldom get sick. My immunity to common viruses has increased. Before, I would catch what was going around the office. I am grateful to Marina for this increased sense of wellbeing and health.

Michelle Ma, Lawyer at Klein Lyons Firm.
Vancouver, British Columbia

How Marina and the Oils Have Impressed Health Professionals . . .

The modern health care consumer is seeking to move beyond the boundaries of allopathic medicine alone, to embrace the healing gifts of nature. With her truly unique intuitive knowledge of the healing power of botanical aromatic essences, Marina expands beyond allopathic practice to offer a highly effective more diverse, holistic healing approach. Her unrivalled intuitive gifts are offered as a remarkable adjunct to, rather than a replacement of, allopathic practice.

Ursula McGarry, MD, Ontario, Canada

I had the chance to meet Marina when she came to Stavanger, Norway in 2009 to share her amazing knowledge and give massages not only to us, but also to others in our community. She graciously took the time to travel all the way from Canada to give my wife and I needed relief in a very hectic part of our lives. Immediately I felt her positive energy and her way of making you feel relaxed and important as a human being. We were going to become proud parents of twins and in addition to that we were working long hours at our busy private eye clinic.

Marina gave us aromatherapy sessions and introduced the essential oils to us, resulting in us being able to manage our high stress levels at the time. Her new book is her own "newborn" and I am looking forward to absorbing her knowledge and positively transforming a lot of our family's current habits for the better. Finally we will be able to enjoy the Aromatherapy Secrets for Wellness at home and learn new ways of dealing with different ailments by using her methods. Our family as well as others she has touched are delighted to have her coming back to Norway in 2012.

Kaare Vigander, Ophthalmologist
ØYELEGENE AS, Stavanger, Norway

I met and trained Marina many years ago in one of the holistic modalities that she mentions in this book. At that time I found Marina's dedication, passion and willingness to learn

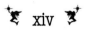

most unique and refreshing to witness.

I am honored and delighted to read her masterpiece of love, devotion and simplicity in facilitating healing for others in this book. She has done it again—this time combining her years of service, experience, knowledge with her excitement that is easy enough to utilize for everyone.

Marina captures the essence of her Divine mission in bearing her soul's journey of passion along with the use of the essences, or 'souls,' of the plants. Her book is easy to read, delightful and practical. Her love for what she does with aromas—essential oils—is very much evidenced throughout her book. I thank you Marina for your wonderful book of aromatherapy that addresses many of today's current problems. Your heart is so pure and caring as it shines in your book. May you the reader enjoy this joy-filled treasure.

Sabina M. DeVita Ed.D. DNM, NNCP, OSJ,
Author of _Electromagnetic Pollution, Saving Face_
& other books
Holistic Practitioner, President, Institute of Energy
Wellness Studies & DeVita Wellness Clinic
Brampton, Ontario Canada

There was a time when our health and healing was achieved and maintained by using natural methods and products. For many years, we have strayed from this way of living, only to find our body, mind and spirit overloaded with toxins, screaming in pain and saddled with stress and its related diseases. It is encouraging to see the use of plant essential oils resuming their rightful place in the story of natural health. These incredibly powerful gifts from Mother Nature are easy, effective and delightful to use.

Marina has made it possible for everyone to naturally achieve comfort, peace and joy through the use of essential oils. Thank you, Marina, for making the world aromatically beautiful again!

Pat Antoniak RN., BN., RA., EOT., AG. Reg.
Registered Nurse – Registered Aromatherapist
Natural Comfort Wellness Centre
Delta, BC. Canada
www.naturalcomfort.ca

Anyone who's had the privilege of spending a few minutes around Marina knows how contagious her energy can be. Her story is one that will inspire anyone seeking to enjoy more health and vitality. From timeless aromatherapy to space age technology, she has information to help anyone achieve wellness beyond his or her dreams.

I have been blessed with her friendship and had the pleasure of sharing her gifts and journey towards health. Read this book and allow yourself to reach for the STARS while smiling from ear to ear!

Eric Groleau
www.GlobalWellnessMedia.com
Ontario, Canada

I first met Marina in 2001 when she came to me as a client. One of my gifts in helping people lies in reading the soul's blueprint and helping people recognize and realize their true soul's potential. During that first session I told her she was going to write a book to help women to use natural modalities to nurture themselves. Over the years since our first meeting Marina has done the arduous inner work necessary to truly fulfill her divine mission, and this book is a must read for anyone desiring to live life to their higher potential. One of the impressions I remember about our first meeting was the amazing vitality and enthusiasm for life that was pouring out of every cell of her being. Marina is a truly passionate, devoted, trustworthy and clear advocate for the profound benefits of aromatherapy. She is a true, insightful and compassionate healer.

Kadea Metara, Catalyst for Change
Spiritual Mentor
Sacramento, California
Kadea.org

"My experience with Marina and her amazing talent for blending essential oils is truly a joy and pleasure. Her love and knowledge of essential oils and her incredible energy is a true gift. There is no doubt in my mind that her book reflects all of this and more!"

Debby Brouwer, Bio Energy Healing Practitioner
http://www.perfecthealth-bioenergy.com/

If only the medical world embraced the healing powers of essential oil… We use, recommend, and sell these "magickal" oils at our shop with amazing results. Calming, healing, energizing- seems to me they do it all!

I have also had the pleasure of receiving aromatherapy massages from my sea sister, Marina Mermaid. All I can say is "total bliss!"

Lynn Carter
Owner, Utopia—The Mystical Sanctuary
North Vancouver
B.C. Canada

Marina Mermaid is a holistic pit-stop for ultimate relaxation with aromatherapy massages and detox treatments. In

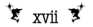

particular, I love her hand-made, chemical-free aromatherapy products. My house and body smell like the south of France – beautiful lavender fields!! Marina is an amazing catalyst for better health and relaxation. Long life to her new book!

Whitney McMillan
Author of *Rock Your Overwhelm: Live in Clarity,*
Balance and Freedom
www.whitneymcmillan.com

Massages can be obtained from a plethora of providers globally…How ever, there is only one person, Marina, with hands so magically intense that can virtually dissolve every ache and pain, and melt you into a fluffy marshmallow state of euphoria. Your book is the true messenger for your passion for aromatherapy.

Caren McSherry
Author, TV host, Chef
Owner, The Gourmet Warehouse
www.thegourmetwarehouse.com

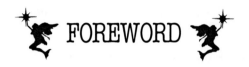

FOREWORD

Marina the Mermaid Makes a Splash

I met Marina several years ago at an aromatherapy retreat. She was radiant, bubbling with energy, and always up for enjoying life to the fullest. It is no surprise to me that *Aromatherapy Secrets for Wellness* is her new creation. Reading through the chapters, I realized that the book is just like her! The writing is warm and comforting, and also full of invaluable information on aromatherapy, essential oils and healing. The prose flows just like her endless energy and it makes you laugh, think, learn and cry.

Working as an aromatherapist, gardener and intuitive healer for the past 15 years my world is dominated by aromas, herbals, plants, seeds, fresh extracts, and oils everywhere. I praise Marina for transforming the world of aromatherapy by giving the essential oils descriptions they truly deserve: essential oils are "like little nurses… and medicine gurus" Absolutely. The oils inspire and heal at the same time. The oils change with time, just like you and I.

In this wonderful aromatic journey through Marina's life and her essential oil teachings, you will discover the fire within you. Her life journey will educate you and draw you into a world of natural healing. The chapter on Stress is of outmost importance in our society. We are stressed and overworked. As Marina writes we have a "strong inability to care for ourselves." Essential oils help you connect, and "set the intention that you are in charge of your own healing."

Are you ready to begin your healing journey? This book will guide you on your way. Enjoy.

Monika Meulman, Hon. BSc. CAHP
The Healing Muse™
Aromatherapist & Intuitive Healer
President of Canadian Federation of Aromatherapists
www.cfacanada.com

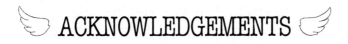

ACKNOWLEDGEMENTS

Waves of Gratitude

To my Family Pillars:

Grand-maman Yvette et ma Tante Suzanne, my guardian angels in heaven.

My papa Pierre Dufort and maman Pierrette Masse, my stepmom Huguette and my stepdad Nounourse (Yves), my brothers Philippe and Guillaume, my sisters Claude and Loulou. Also their precious partners Anahi, Myriam, Michou (mayor of Skidoune Ville) and Dodo (Gazebo). And a warm welcome to my one-week old niece, Adèle Dufort.

My mother in law Marie-Claire (Petite Ecureuil) and all my hilarious aunts, uncles and cousins from the Masse and Dufort families. You know who you are!

To my Book Birth Pillars:

From Coquitlam, British Columbia, Bob Burnham, my mentor, author and publisher who lives in a bunker—his office is totally drama proof—and creates miracles repeatedly. Merci Bob.

From New York to Los Angeles, Rosemary Sneeringer, my precious Doula Editor who gets the words out magically, using a lot of humour and spiritual essences to smooth out the process of writing and creating your own true book. I bow to you sister. All right then!

In Philadelphia, Susan Veach, the Queen of book cover imaging and concepting, a fabulous graphic artist who literally nailed it. Merci Susan.

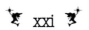

In Denver, Colorado, Rebecca Hanna, the magician designer for the esthetics of my book.

In Chicago, Illinois, Alison Howard, my meticulous, detail-oriented proofreader.

Thanks to Lee Halliday Photography for the atomizer picture on the cover.

To my Heart to Heart Pillar:

Jean Michel for the last 13 years of companionship. Merci c'est gentil!

To my Aromatherapy Pillars:

Pat Antoniak, my first teacher and mentor. My CFA sisters and president Monika Meulman. My BCAOA and BCAPA aroma sisters.

All my aromatherapy clients from the film industry. Rob McLachlan, my dear friend. My regulars and my clients at Women's Retreats with Heather at Loon Lake, now dear friends.

To my Wellness Leaders and Pillars:

Janine Brolly, my Sunshine sister. Nicole and Rob Stewart, my rocks of Excellence. Ashley Stewart, the nine-year-old spiritual angel of the group. Thanks to all the miracle stories from my friends and clients rebuilding their health with the best nutritional cleansing products out there, I am forever your biggest fan and wellness cheerleader.

To my Beauty Pillars:

Jacqueline Couture-Brisdon, Tami Esau, Yuki Arndt. Kelly Siegmann, my hair-apist who also did my hair and make up for the picture on my back cover! Cher Anderson, my sea sister and designer of the amazing necklace on my back cover picture. Marie-Lyne Denomme and Marie-Jeanne Godard. Je t'aime!

To my Spiritual Pillars:

The Girls of Utopia, Farhad Khan, Jen Jordan, Debbie Brouwer, Eric & Annie. Nicola and Scot McDonald at Full Frame productions, who took my picture for the back cover. My Equinox Circle, we are 29 members with our fairy leader Doreen Virtue. Love you so much!

To my Financial Pillars:

Sam Harris and Christian White, Directors at Investors Group, who taught me how to get organized with my prosperity. Priceless!

To my National and International Mermaids Sea Sisters and Merman Pillars:

All my dears friends, mentors, teachers, inspirational souls that I have connected with during my passionate pilgrimage through life, a big heart-to-heart hug!

TO MY GUIDES AND ANGELS AND MALE ELVES, SOLDIERS OF LOVE

Merci De tout Coeur xxx

Marina Mermaid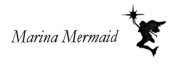

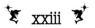

DISCLAIMER

It is very important for you to consult a doctor before making changes in your diet and lifestyle and before using essential oils or taking vitamin and/or food supplements. While care has been taken gathering and presenting the information in this book, the author accepts neither liability nor responsibility to any person with respect to loss, injury, and damage caused or alleged, as the direct or indirect result of the information contained in this book.

The purpose of this book is to educate and inform. For medical advice you should seek the individual, personal services of a medical professional.

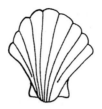

Step into my world of relaxation. Live vicariously through an essential oil treatment with Marina . . .

The first moment your foot touches the path, your journey has begun. You feel a calmness as you step on pebbles mixed with Zen garden stones surrounded by grass, lavender plants and flowers. Opening the door, the mists of pure Pine or Sweet Orange essential oils lets your brain know you are already in the zone for rejuvenation. Marina greets you with a big smile and a heart-to-heart hug. You hear the water in the Romanesque fountain and smell the cleansing smells of nature, as the subdued light and candles welcome you into the soft seashell of her caring hands. After having completed your Wellness data sheet and discussed it with Marina you are now ready.

The massage room is clear, full of light and love just for you. The music is soothing with nature sounds to connect you with Mother Earth, Goddess of Heart and Home. Everything is in place for maximum relaxation. Now you decide your main intention or purpose for your session today so you can have a blissful experience.

The temperature is always warm. Colors are white, pale purple and *café au lait*. Orchids are everywhere. The massage table is covered in gold velvet sheets or fresh clean flannel with plush comforters. Marina calls it the "Rocking Gondola," large and comfortable.

You are told which of the 11 oils will be used with the warm carrier oil of your choice—Apricot Kernel oil, Evening Primrose, or Rosehips oil. The essential oils are enhanced by the use of warm river rocks and volcanic or jade stones. The signature Marina Mermaid Session uses Derma Ray Jade Esthetics, a high frequency electrotherapy device developed by Dr. Charles McWilliams. Referred to as a "cellular massage," it improves circulation and increases your energy level, while elevating the oxygen in your blood. This device helps push the blend of oils more efficiently into your metabolism, so you feel refreshed.

The signature session comes complete with Shiatsu, Swedish, Reflexology, Lymphatic Drainage, Thigh Brushing and Abdomen Soak (your choice of five: Constipation (❀ *Flow*), Heartburn (❀ *Digestive Warrior*), Gas (❀ *Belly Zen*), Food poisoning (❀ *Detox: The Cleaner*), or Parasites (❀ *Parasites Me? No Way*) for your digestive system, if needed. All of this is blissfully accomplished in a 90-minute session.

To release toxins after the session, the finest Ionic Footbath on the market is an option. Afterward, it's time to hydrate with lemon, cucumber or orange water. You get the luscious treat of green tea chocolate loaded with minerals to help rebalance your sugar levels. After an aromatherapy session, your body continues to release toxins for up to 24 hours, so plenty of water is suggested.

At the close of the session, you're feeling grounded in your body, relaxed, positive and more connected to what's important in your life. The book *Sick and Tired* by Dr. Robert O. Young is recommended. It discusses essential alkalinity for health. On the alkalinity/acidity scale in your stomach, lemon becomes +9.9 and cucumber becomes +31.5. Beef is -34.5.

Then we talk about how you feel and what you would like to improve for the next session. You are offered the perfect healing oils for you to recreate your spa experience at home...

What a difference from what I could sense when you entered my studio!

Here's how my Signature Marina Mermaid Sessions transform lives:

- I can feel you on your way before you get here
- I hear your high heels tapping and your voice on your mobile phone giving last-minute orders to your employees
- I sense your internal stress from work

I take your coat, your briefcase, you armor, getting you ready to be relaxed on the table. You are usually out of breath, sweaty, stressed out and accustomed to moving fast. When you enter, you are relieved—your breathing pattern shifts. I offer you water, invite you to use the restroom, to remove your clothes and put on a nice fresh robe. Then I ask for a brief explanation of what you are looking for in a session. What is your focus or intention today? This helps maximize your time with me.

Sometimes men will come in, hunched over, sent in by their wives. They don't want to be here. After the session, they don't have to hide the fact that they like aromatherapy. "I can still

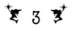

feel some pain, and my phone's ringing, but I still feel so much better now," they'll say. "Now I see why my wife likes coming here." After the session they are like jelly and have a big loopy grin. I tell them to look in the mirror and see their souls. I suggest using the oils at home—every time you take a whiff you will remember your session with Marina. It stimulates the limbic system, the ancient brain, processing center of your reason, your instinct, your emotions and sense of smell. They say they realize they need to take time for themselves and ask when they can come back.

Sessions raise the client's frequency. Their eyes are rested, the pupils are dilated, and the whites are lighter and less yellow. After a massage, their bodies are more alkaline. They may be thirsty for the next few days, as the kidneys and liver will be cleaning out. It's a pleasant way to detox. If you have a glass of wine or champagne, this is how you feel after a session with me.

Many times the clients don't recognize the health benefits before they come in. A session with me cracks the door open to shift people into wellness, into taking care of themselves. I tell them to drink a lot of water, even if they don't like it. They breathe more deeply afterward and raise their oxygen levels. Endorphin levels are higher and their cortisol levels drop.

The changes I have seen in the life of my steady clients are enormous:

- They start to line up things that need to be changed

- They feel like they need to slow down, even if they are successful in business

- They take more time for themselves and for aromatherapy and massage

- They are not as stressed as they were

- They take up hobbies or go on adventures out of their comfort zones

- They put themselves first on the list—shift the hierarchy

- They are able to work more with less stress

- They let go of negative relationships

- They grieve and move on

- They become more clear about what they want in life

- They become the leader of the pack

When I first began my practice, I attracted people with a lot of drama in their lives because I had a lot of drama in mine. Now I have regulars who are deeply connected to themselves.

My clients tell me that at work they can now change their focus and become more productive. They begin to excel in their professions, even after making their own wellness a priority. They start to think more positively. They say "no" more and deliver better quality. They manage their time better, hire assistants, and progress in their careers. Mediocrity becomes a thing of the past.

Many lose weight once they make themselves number one, especially working moms. They are challenged for time with all the things they do for their kids—taxi moms taking children to ballet, karate, soccer, hockey, painting, school activities, and working to pay for all of it. Sometimes they bring their kids in for relaxation, because they are overachievers and stressed too. I want to work on the whole family—even the dog. I've made special blends for animals. It helps the collective family feel better and get along better. I am proud to be part of my clients' lives and I care about their achievements. I encourage them and cheer them on! I really feel like their Personal Wellness Cheerleader.

And now I'm making these benefits available to you in your own home…

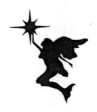

I've always been fascinated by mermaids and their playfulness. Cher Anderson hand made this mermaid necklace for me.

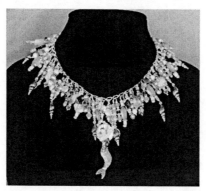

Cher and I met in San Diego and developed a wonderful relationship based on our mutual love of Mermaids. "*Mermaid at Play*," a wonderful painting by Cher, can also be viewed on my website at: www.marinamermaid.com/mermaidatplay

Cher is the Founder of Cher's Creations, LLC from where she designs and sells original necklaces and artwork. She specializes in one-of-a-kind designs with natural stones and gems from all over the world.

The synergy developed between Marina Mermaid and I is as natural as that of gems and essential oils, the Angels of our Mother Earth.

All my best,
Cher
Cher Anderson, Founder of Cher's Creations, LLC
www.cherscreations.com
Arizona, USA

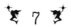

*There are two mistakes one can
make along the road to truth... Not
going all the way, and not starting.*
  -Buddha

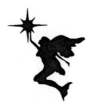

The Marina Mermaid Story

I was born under the sign of Fire Horse, the 18th of April 1966. My name is Marie Yvette Nathalie Masse Dufort. The name Masse is the verb "massaging" and Dufort means "strong." Funny that even my name advertised my passion in this life.

For many years when I was a kid I had a recurring dream of being trapped under a big medieval door where villagers placed heavy stones until I suffocated to death. I later found out that in medieval times, marriages were pre-arranged between families at birth. A girl born under Fire Horse was simply considered too rebellious, independent and hard to control, so these female babies were drowned.

Since I was a little girl, I had this fear in my heart of being ostracized, fear of being attacked, fear of being different. As a kid I just knew that I had some special gifts. I felt much older and with much more wisdom than other kids. I knew that the older we got, the more we would forget this wisdom. I had an open heart and wanted to share all I had. I got in trouble for this several times. Once I wrote the answers in a schoolmate's notebook and he got in trouble for cheating. His big brother came to school and pushed me against the wall with his hands around my neck and told me not to help his brother any more. I always knew that I had been killed and silenced many times in past lives for my desire to help people heal in other lives. I made the promise to myself when I was seven years old never to become an adult—a blind and boring adult. And I have kept that kid part of me alive. Kids see and feel and know so much. I want people to be aware of their precious wisdom.

I grew up in the Province of Quebec and I can still smell the scents I experienced as a four year old roaming the mini-garden and enchanted forest of cedar, cypress and pine that belonged to my Grand-papa Eugene Dufort and my Grand-maman Berthe. This was a family of five baby girls and my daddy, Pierre Dufort, was the only man in that tribe. The house was <u>huge</u> to me and as a child I ventured forth and used my nose to investigate. During one visit I took all the decorative mini-savonettes in each bathroom and hid them in my little bag. Why? I was fascinated with flowery fragrances and aromas.

I was very serious about proper observance of commemorative rituals, almost like a Vestal in charge of the sacred fire and keeper of natural remedies during the Roman Empire. When I was five, I found a dead bird on our front lawn and I covered the poor thing with a white tissue, then gathered all the kids on the block to make sure he had a proper funeral with songs to send him to the afterworld. This instinct was stronger than me, this fascination with the proper, respectful way to do things, and I was deeply touched by death.

I was allowed to drink my first glass of red wine (mixed with water) and I felt so lucky to be granted that ceremony of sharing the wine and the bread with those who love you. Thanks to my so cool parents of the seventies!

When I was seven, we lived in Sept-Iles and my father was the manager of the Employment Centre of Canada. He was hired to help Native Americans find work and keep their dignity with government programs. We lived in a big white house near the Indian Reservation, and I knew the kids were poor. In my heart I thought that I was helping them by hiding 15 of them, between four and seven years old, in my closet, aided by a big bag of teddy bear lollypops to keep them quiet and happy with me, the rich Caucasian girl. I thought they could live there, no problem. When they were discovered during dinnertime, my parents were horrified. We could have been sued for kidnapping! I just wanted them to forget about their own lives for few hours…

I also learned that we were not going to hang out forever on planet Earth. My favorite family member was my Grand-maman Yvette. Once when she was visiting us, I asked her casually during dinner, "Are you going to stay in this human form forever grand-maman?" Big silence. Then she told me she would die some day. Wow, I just could not wrap that idea around my little head. I was in trauma and I started to cry. My dad had to take me away in my room and hold me in his arms while I sobbed away. He was trying to calm me down, but I just did not want to accept the idea of not being here anymore. I thought we humans were all immortals. In my heart I knew we were all souls and lived forever, but now my parents were telling me, no, you will die too. That made me very angry.

We finally moved near my grandparents Yvette and Pitou in Berthierville. I felt so lucky to be reunited with Yvette. At eight years old, she was driving me to the Catholic Church. I was so small but I remember the plastic Virgin Mary glued to the dashboard of her big gold Buick. I enjoyed this amazing quality time with her. The silence we shared in the church during the frankincense ritual was heaven to me. What a great way to get high legally as a child. This was the best time of my life. I loved that smell because it symbolized love and peace and protection. Grand-maman smelled like sugar mixed with lavender and frankincense to me.

As a kid I was always asking family and guests if I could massage their backs or hands and I used to walk on my father's back to release his spine tension. At ten, I was already devouring a lot of books and had learned the basic meaning of the lines on the palms, *la chiromancie*. Before we took the bus to school in the morning I read my friends' hands to kill time. Not the usual type of activity for a kid my age…

Elementary school was so painful for me. The kids were so mean. I loved learning. I was skinny and tall. I knew I was a nerd, but I was an artistic nerd.

I was in love with a little boy named Andre Desjardin. I recall helping arrange soft drink glass bottles in our Masse family grocery/gas station. I was carrying a case of empty bottles when my knees went numb and I smelled Andre. I knew he came to say *"Adieu mon amie."* He had just passed.

A few minutes later, a customer entered our store and told my family that this little boy, Andre Desjardin, just got killed on his bike by a driver. Of course I did not say anything about his goodbye, but I knew. At school the next day I brought a red rose and put it on his desk.

I will never forget the funeral service. The smell of his little embalmed body and his little swollen face covered in makeup is so imprinted on my brain. The week before, the whole school had gone to church for another funeral. Someone in my class had an older brother who died and Andre said to me, "I am so young, there is no way I could die now!" He was laughing. I guess I was the lucky one who felt his presence. God bless Andre.

For my 16th birthday, Grand-maman Yvette gave me my first suitcase and said, "Travel, be free and enjoy life, do not stay here. Live your Freedom." And so did I! I left home at 16. I was on the leash no more! My mom paid for my modest bachelor apartment so I could study French Literature in college. I really wanted to be an actress. I was getting life experience under the belt so I could be accepted in a great theatre school.

At 18 years old I took my first introductory massage therapy class at the University of Montreal and I was hooked! A few years later I completed my Bachelors in Drama at the University of Quebec in Montreal. I was 26 when Grand-maman Yvette got snatched away by cancer on June 7, 1992. She came to me during my sleep and did a funky maneuver over my body with her great soul, and gave me a last huge warm hug of pure love. The phone rang. It was my stepdad, Nounourse, who only said "It is done."

That last visit from her gave me the boost to write her eulogy that I read in "our" Church of Berthierville, and again the frankincense aroma comforted me while I followed her big blue steel casket outside of the church. The bells sang so loud to me... Ding dong time is ticking, ding dong time to go, ding dong time for your mission...

My blood, the wise woman who gave me strength and always held me dear, was gone. I was numb and deaf and sodden with grief. I looked for her everywhere. I read so many books on life after death to find out where she went. Even Edgar Cayce could not calm me down. I was living in Plateau Mont-Royal, in Montreal, where I found a little metaphysical store. I bought jade stones to ground myself, essential oils and incense. In my dark green room with brick walls and candles, I indulged myself in pine, cedar, cypress, spruce and frankincense oils— the aromatic balm of my childhood.

I came to understand the power of having a comforting spiritual sanctuary to heal my soul. I was able to connect with my pain and finally start to let it go. I was embarking on my spiritual quest and the essentials oils became my little nurses and personal therapists and medicinal gurus for so many ailments. I was finally home. I became a Soldier of Love.

At that time, I was working on TV shows. I had done theatre, traveled in many countries, had been in many relationships, and in too many snowstorms to count. I was ready to spread my wings. In April 1995 I left Quebec in a '68 Chevy Van to cross Canada and start my new life in Banff and find my authentic self. My name was Marie-Nathalie Dufort, "Gypsy Mermaid of the Rockies." (This story is available in *Change One Belief*, an anthology compiled by Bob Burnham, by Expert Author Publishing.)

While this is a mystical, soul-driven account of my childhood and the growth of my spirit, there is another side to my growing up years—the physical side, which I came to understand, was directly related to my emotional life. That is why sitting in the little room in Plateau Mont-Royal was so powerful, because I found the keys to heal my heart, which healed my body and sealed my fate as a healer of many. Indeed, I am only the messenger.

I want you to know, dear reader, that I have been in your shoes. Over the years I have been overweight, with high cholesterol and repeated tonsil infections. After having my tonsils extracted, my immune system was compromised, giving me allergies, hay fever and bronchitis.

I was born with scoliosis and I had many pains and aches in my back since childhood. I had constipation—just ask my whole family! I basically lived in the bathroom. My poor sister

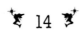

had to hold our school bus almost every morning because I was stuck in the washroom! I was also a sugar addict and an avid junk food consumer—the family grocery business fed this habit. I had problems with circulation and I was an insomniac. I was a super sensitive case study! Oh, and I also was a smoker for 6 years!

Well, well, well. Thank God for aromatherapy in my life. The gradual use and discovery of the oils, and my studies over the years, have made me so much healthier and stronger. Now I am rarely sick or have discomfort.

My mission now is to help you connect to the essential oils, and I believe that if you do just that, your body and soul are going undergo a huge transformational experience. You will finally get out of the situation (emotional, mental, spiritual, physical) you have been in for too long. I am talking here about a profound liberating flowing wave of wellness and a huge kick of self-love in your human electrical frequencies. My second book, already in the works, is talking about healing modalities to help you to reach this higher level of wellness.

I am personally an essential oil addict and proud to be. I am high on the oils. I am high on life. I am high on love.

After I took my first massage therapy course at the University of Montreal, I became a trained TV and radio host and actor (Bachelor in Drama from the University of Quebec in Montreal), and a member of Union des Artistes in Quebec. I am also a trained film industry professional, a member of the Union of British Columbia Performers and a member of the Alliance of Canadian Cinema, Television and Radio Artists.

Having established myself in front of the cameras in my twenties, I felt a big void inside of me. While at first it had

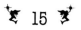

been so interesting, I was bored. I lost my passion for talking about other actors or artists. Even though I was famous and getting paid to be on TV, something was missing. After my grand-maman's death, the West Coast of Canada was pulling me to where I could blossom with my gifts. I worked in a bohemian little bar called The Gypsy Club where a Parisien psychic told me I would have a life shift into holistic studies and aromatherapy massages. I resisted the idea for so long, not believing in myself. Then having made the move to Banff for a year, I traveled to Vancouver for a visit, and a friend living in Japan knew I was between jobs. She said, "Marina, it is the perfect time for you to make a change." She sent me a one-way ticket to Osaka and said I could pay her back whenever I got the money. I traveled to Japan. Ultimately, I spent two years there studying massage, and have never stopped learning since.

In two weeks, I found a job teaching English with cue cards to Japanese pre-school kids. I got an apartment with three Canadian roommates. I had a headache and a friend who was going to school for Shiatsu pressed my hand and in three minutes got rid of a migraine I had for two days. I was blown away and decided to study acupressure in Japan.

Here are the results of the studies I threw myself into:

- Studied Shiatsu at The Cohrin Academy of Shiatsu in Osaka, Japan

- Certified Aromatherapy Health Professional (CAHP)

- Registered Aromatherapist (R.A.)

- Essential Oil Therapist (E.O.T.)

- Member of National CFA (Canadian Federation of Aromatherapists)

- Member of BCAOA (British Columbia Association of Aromatherapists)

- Member of BCAPA (British Columbia Alliance of Practicing Aromatherapists)

- Derma Ray Therapist trained by Dr Sabina M. de Vita, author of *Electromagnetic Pollution* and founder of the Institute of Energy and Wellness Studies in Ontario.

- Lymphatic Drainage Practitioner

- Certified Reflexologist by Touch Point Canadian Institute of Reflexology in British Columbia

- Jade Stone Massage Therapist

- Certified Chair Massage Practitioner

- Ear Candling Detox Practitioner

I have been massaging cast and crew in the film industry, as well as music industry clients, since 1997. I enjoy working with people who are ready for a change in their lives. I have introduced aromatherapy and massages to 10,000 people so far.

I can help you to move forward from physical discomfort and emotional stress to radiant health and wellbeing with the simple use of sacred essential oils in your daily life. My desire is to share the healing properties of aromatherapy so that everyone can benefit. I give you my recipes and blends freely, hoping you will find health and wellbeing, and become happier and more balanced.

You may find that, like a painter or any kind of artist, you'll begin to make your own blends and discover that it's not that complicated—it's just a matter of trusting your nose and finding your favorite concoctions. My goal is to help people open up the door to their creativity with the use of essential oils, not to make them dependent on me.

My passion for holistic wellbeing in the last 25 years has given me extensive experience in the field of making people proactive in their <u>own</u> healing. My ultimate goal is to make you feel better by reaching total bliss and harmony with your body, your temple. Then the magic happens. When the temple is at peace, the mind and spirit and emotions are also unified in love and light, creating higher vibrations ready to elevate you to your pure potential.

You are blessed, and my job is to treat you like a pearl you already are in the seashell of my caring hands...

Marina Dufort, Mermaid of Holistic Aromatherapy, November 2011

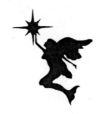

*Accept the fact that some days
you're the pigeon, and some days
you're the statue!*
-Unknown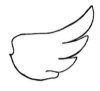

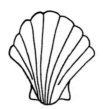

Seashell #1
How the Oils Transform Struggle and Dissolve Stress

Stress is like this little hamster on steroids scratching the walls of your cortex trying to get out. The famous Mayo Clinic for medical education says that stress is what you experience when the level of your stressors exceeds your ability to cope. To lower your stress level, you have two options. Option *numéro un* is to identify the sources of your stress that you can then eliminate. Internal stressors include fears and unrealistic expectations. External strategies for coping with stress include relaxation techniques, aromatherapy, exercising, music, creativity and humor. Option *numéro deux* is to simplify your life by saying "no."

Often the main motivation to go to a spa or to meet with a holistic practitioner is to relieve stress. Did you know that 50% of clients come for a relaxation session to deal with a high level of stress and 38% of spa-goers are looking for relief for sore joints or sore muscles? The paradigm of the spa industry is undergoing a big shift: the industry is moving from pampering to wellness, and stress management has become its new philosophy.

Stress is the silent killer. We need stress to get ourselves up in the morning and meet with life. This is positive stress. But when the stress builds up because of a feeling of danger— when you think you are in emotional or physical peril—your mind is concerned with whether you are able to deal with the urgent situation or not, and your body pumps adrenaline into your system. This is the fight-or-flight response. If the adrenaline boost is not used on a physical level, the adrenaline stays in your body, creating tension and emotional distress. When we build up too much stress without relief, we become strained, drained, tense, irritable and so tired. Sound familiar? We are bombarded by constant demands and expectations. We all have our triggers or our sensitivities. I'm talking here about situational stress.

Common causes of situational stress are losing someone or something important, dealing with family and relationship issues, holding negative attitudes, having health problems and financial insecurities, feeling powerless and uncertain about the future, interacting with negative people, fearing failure, experiencing job-related issues, coping with low self-esteem and feeling responsible for everyone or everything.

When too much is too much, all of this situational stress will create allergies, asthma, anger, cardiovascular disease, digestive problems, high blood pressure, heart disease, inefficient action, inability to think clearly, increased errors, insomnia, migraines, headaches, mild depression, premature aging, tension, anxiety, ulcers, skin problems, obesity and more.

If you feel like a Chihuahua on the edge, there is a good chance your mind and body are under attack by stress in your daily life. It is as if your natural alarm system is constantly on. Every time you perceive a threat, your hypothalamus gland sets off the alarm system in your body, through the nerves and hormonal system, causing your adrenals to release hormones, including adrenaline and cortisol. Cortisol increases blood sugar, suppresses the immune system and decreases bone formation.

Human bodies are so wonderful. The human body has an amazing ability for adaptation. However, the more easily we can adapt to the pressures around us, the greater our temptation to push ourselves beyond our limits. Stress is very insidious; it deforms our thinking. After a while we believe it is normal to be stressed out. We adapt. We push and we push and we push until one day, our bodies put the brakes on and say "enough," and we find ourselves with an unwanted condition. Did you know that 80% of medical consultations are prompted by stress? The root of this is a strong inability to care for ourselves.

That's why I love aromatherapy, the therapy that makes use of essential oils and causes little or no side effects. It is an art and a science of using essential oils for improving and maintaining your health and your beauty. With aromatherapy in your life, you can switch your stress from a level ten (super over-the-top, terrible crying-out-loud painful) to a lower level—the peace level, the breathable and livable level. Aromatherapy is an excellent tool against stress. When you are inhaling essential oils, you are asserting that you are in charge of your own healing. Over time, your wonderfully adaptive body will learn a different stress response and will thank you for it.

Because essential oils contain highly concentrated plant properties, they are able to treat a number of ailments. When you breathe in the oils, they stimulate various psychological and physical responses. When they are massaged into the skin, tiny oil particles pass into the body and are utilized. Signals are passed directly to the limbic system in the brain, provoking an immediate emotional or instinctual response. The amygdala is fantastic for that. The almond-shaped amygdalae are located in your medial temporal lobes (called your limbic system) and are responsible for processing all your cellular memories, good and bad, and your emotional reactions. They also serve as the center for reason and smell. The olfactory system is so powerful.

The use of scent in healing has been highly underestimated. Essential oils are little angels ready to protect you as soon as you ask for their help and support. I believe in the power of essential oils, they are as magical to me as my favorite American shows I watched as a kid, *I Dream of Jeannie*, *Bewitched* and *The Flying Nun*.

Stress occurs from fixating on both the past and the future, telling yourself, "I should have done this or that," or, "When I will be rich I will be stress-free. When I will be perfect I will be stress-free. When I will be free I will be stress-free." As the British would say… "Bullocks! I am <u>now</u>!"

Negative emotional patterns can stem from orienting yourself in the future. Instead of "When I will," the oils bring you into "I am now." Instead of saying, "When I will be rich I will be stress- free," try saying, "I am now rich. I am now perfect, I am now stress-free."

With the help of my British friend Sam Harris Ba (Hons) and Division Director at Investors Group, I was able to work on my financial stress reprogramming. My mindset is now in the right state. I also helped Sam to incorporate regular holistic sessions in his lifestyle.

"The Investment business can be stressful on the mind and body. Many have relieved my stresses in the past, but no one comes close to the dexterity and skill of Marina Dufort.

After leaving her clinic for the first time, I was so relaxed, I couldn't drive!

What makes Marina unique is her in-depth understanding of the mind and body both in terms of physicality and spirituality.

After an hour on her table I can take on the world.

Bring it on...."

"Marina Dufort is the most accomplished Aromatherapist on the West Coast of North America. Her dexterity is unprecedented in lowering the stress levels of any patient"

"There are few world class Aromatherapists - Marina Dufort is one of them."

"I have experienced Aromatherapy in many places including Europe, Russia and North America. Marina Dufort is the shining star and worth crossing any continent for."

Sam Harris.

I want to make sure you understand the power of synergy. The term "synergy" comes from the Greek word syn-ergos, meaning working together. When you are using one single essential oil alone, it is helpful, but if you mix two or three or more together, then you are making the effect so much more powerful. As Valerie Ann Worwood says in *The Complete Book of Essential Oils & Aromatherapy*, "When the combination is more than the sum of the parts, there is a synergistic effect. By mixing together two or more essential oils you are creating a chemical compound that is different to any of the component parts, and these synergistic blends are very particular and powerful... they enhance each other..."

Now I will take you on a journey through the mind, heart and nose, the laboratory of this aromatherapist. We are going to create a stress-buster blend. This peek behind my curtain will demonstrate why I have selected these oils for one of the most important jobs in today's society—to soothe your stress so you can reclaim your wellness.

To do that, this blend needs to meet the following exacting criteria for me and for you. It must be pleasing, happy and uplifting, but also bring you down to earth, into the present moment. It must connect with your heart so you will not "spin" tales of your life into negative outcomes, but rather will be able to create the life you desire from a calm and centered space.

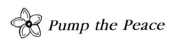

The brand I want to talk to you about is called ❀ *Pump the Peace* blend. It helps you release and let go of tension and anxiety when your stress level is out of control.

FRANKINCENSE

The grounding oil in my ❀ *Pump the Peace* blend is Frankincense for your crown chakra. I use Frankincense because it is "the Windex of your spiritual patio door. The Mister Clean of your third eye." I say that to you so you can visualize the powerful spiritual cleansing effect of this oil when you use it. Forgive me for using chemical commercial brands as examples, but I am convinced that holistic alternatives can do everything the chemical world can do and more, so you can enjoy health and wellbeing in a safe manner.

One of my favorite activities when I was a kid was going to Catholic mass with grand-maman Yvette. I loved it when they would burn the Frankincense incense and cover it with a little cloak. I was eight years old and it was my favorite part of the ceremony. I was told as a five-year-old kid that Frankincense, Gold and Myrrh were the gifts brought by the Three Wise Men to Baby Jesus when he was born. That made me cry with joy. I felt so at peace when I smelled that incense.

Before I became an aromatherapist, I was given a pure chunk of Frankincense resin from my friend Felix who brought it back from Egypt. I burned it with great respect on a small hot charcoal and had amazing answers to my prayers when feeling too anxious. Frankincense has been used since antiquity, in India, China, the Middle East and in the Western World, especially by the Catholic Church. In ancient Egypt it was used in facial masks (the typical Egyptian black thick line under the eyes was made with Frankincense), cosmetics and perfume, and also as part of a purification process. The Pharaohs used essences to control their people, to relax them so they would not become aggressive, and for seduction as well. The use of aromas with religious rituals was very important for pleasing the Gods. Some Egyptians slaves were used as giant incense holders with burning incense cones on their heads.

Uses of Frankincense: It is excellent for relieving mental chatter, frustration, nervous system anxiety, nervous tension and stress-related conditions. It's very sedative and helpful if you have an addiction of some sort, as it will calm you down. It is highly regarded for healing and can stimulate the immune system. Frankincense contains sesquiterpenes that help stimulate the pineal gland, which secretes melatonin, a hormone that enhances deep sleep. It also helps to overcome despair.

David Hoffman, who wrote a book called ✴ *The New Holistic Herbal*, said that Frankincense has among its physical properties the ability to slow down and deepen breath, which is very conducive to prayer and meditation. Frankincense helped me to grieve my Grand-maman Yvette when she lost her battle to cancer. I was able to release old emotional traumas and move on with more peace. For thousands of years, many spiritual practices included the sacred use of this amazing healing essential oil. I feel that Frankincense is the symbolic brother of Archangel Michael in the realm of ✴ "Angel Therapy" taught by sweet Doreen Virtue. I have been sharing her Angel Card messages for the last 6 years. Frankincense oil is like the peaceful warrior of essential oils to help you to empower your physical temple with courage, focus and safety. Combine it with a sacred pure intention with the infinity symbol (∞ the powerful number eight on its side) to propel your frequency to a higher level of healing.

SWEET ORANGE

There is a family of essential oils that is very effective for stress called the *Rutaceae* (botanical family name). This citrus family of essential oils is represented by Bergamot, Grapefruit, Lemon, Lime, Mandarin, Neroli (Orange Blossom), Orange (Bitter), Orange (Sweet), Petitgrain and Tangerine. These oils are your natural antidepressants, antioxidants, and anti-anxiety aids.

For many years I have been spritzing Sweet Orange or Neroli essential oils mixed with water all over myself, in my studio, in my car, on my friends, in my bedroom, on my coworkers— because it works so fast! This is the best uplifter for me. I am very fond of citrus essential oils. They are the twin sisters of your girlish girl kid within or the twin brothers of your internal boyish boy. They can flip your mood instantly, in two seconds from down to peaceful. They are the smiling oils.

Marketing studies reveal that almost anyone who enters a business or a shopping place or an area they aren't familiar with turn right. They do this because they don't know where they are going. Did you know that 99% of people turn right? That's great to know when you're setting up displays of your product. But one of the big breakthrough shockers in marketing research also shows that olfactory senses attract buying customers when Orange essential oils are diffused. People stop and relax and become more open. Customers will be more likely to treat themselves and buy more when breathing Orange and other citrus oils.

Sweet Orange is a very nutritious fruit containing vitamins A B and C. If you want to lower your stress level, use different varieties of citrus. The Chinese love using citrus for that reason. It helps you calm down when too much is happening in your hectic life. Aromatherapy uses for citrus and orange are as sedatives, useful for nervous tension and stress-related conditions, hyperactivity and emotional and mental burnout. It soothes your autonomic nervous system. I enjoy using any of the citrus essential oils to reduce stress levels. When I use citrus oils, I visualize laughing kids. I enjoy asking for the help of Archangel Chamuel, the special angel who attracts personal and global peace in your life. He also helps to raise your love vibrations.

YLANG YLANG

Ylang Ylang. I just love pronouncing the name of this essential oil, it sounds so sexy to me. It has been used to cover beds of newlywed couples on their wedding night, for skin treatments, and for thick, shiny lustrous hair and without split ends. It is also great for regulating the heartbeat and respiration.

Ylang Ylang helps to balance male and female energy. Again, I enjoy working with the help of Archangel Chamuel to help to raise the love vibration for yourself and toward others when using Ylang Ylang. Your people skills will grow more naturally with the use of this oil, and you will connect heart-to-heart more effortlessly.

Aromatherapy uses: Ylang Ylang fights mood swings, anger, depression, anxiety, shock, panic, fear and stress-related conditions. It relieves high blood pressure, calms autistic people and it is good for excitable conditions where the adrenalin is way too elevated. Ylang Ylang is a wonderful aphrodisiac, uplifts sexual energy, and will enhance your relationships. Because it is a calming and relaxing essential oil, it helps with anger and rage and self-esteem issues.

The widely accepted translation of Ylang Ylang is "flower of flowers." The fragrance is rich and deep, with hints of Jasmine and Neroli. It is widely used in perfumery for oriental and floral themed perfumes such as Chanel No.5.

BLENDING ❀ *Pump the Peace*

Mix all three essential oils starting with three drops of Frankincense. Then add your citrus oil, Sweet Orange, the uplifter of your girlish-girl energy or boyish-boy energy. This is your laughing oil. Use six drops. Then add the essential oil Ylang Ylang, which helps to circulate your blood. Use two drops. Mix these essential oils first in an empty 10 ml glass bottle and smell the synergy. Now you are ready to pour the ultimate carrier oil for peace and safety, Jojoba oil, your natural preservative, in your 10 ml glass bottle. Voila!

Pronounced ho-HO-ba, Jojoba is a botanical extract of the seed of the plant *Simmondsia Chinensis*. Technically it's not an oil, but a wax ester. This wax ester is most similar to human skin oil (sebum). It's extracted from the bean of the plant and is a natural preservative. It does not lose its therapeutic qualities even if it solidifies in cold temperatures. When in liquid form it has a rich gold color. It is theorized that applying jojoba to the skin can trick the skin into thinking it is producing enough oil, thus balancing oil production. Jojoba is noncomedogenic as well, which means it does not block pores. The therapeutic properties of jojoba are amazing— it is a natural preservative and an emulsifier, and has both sunscreen and anti-inflammatory qualities. Because jojoba oil has a common saturated fatty acid (myristic acid), it is very gentle and safe to use as a natural eye and makeup remover. It is expensive, but it is a must in your personal carrier oil kit at home. Jojoba is very stable and does not go rancid. When you use this oil there is no contraindication.

And now  **Pump the Peace** is born in your hands, the blend that will help relax you and take you from level ten stress to seven, six, five, four or three with each different application.

Pump the Peace

Application: Inhale or use as a perfume. Mix 15 drops of the blend in a water bottle spritzer and spritz and inhale when needed.

<u>Frankincense</u>. Base note, grounding. Botanical name: *Boswellia carteri* from the botanical family *Burseraceae*.

Safety Data: Non-toxic, non-irritant.

<u>Sweet Orange</u>. Top note, very uplifting. Botanical Name: *Citrus sinensis* from the botanical family *Rutaceae*.

Safety Data: Generally non-toxic. Can cause skin irritation in those with sensitive skin and photosensitivity. Avoid exposure to direct sunlight if you have had a massage with this oil.

<u>Ylang Ylang</u>. Base note, very grounding. Botanical Name: *Cananga odorata* from the botanical family *Annonaceae*.

Safety Data: Non-toxic, non-irritant. Use in moderation since its heady scent can cause headaches or nausea if you inhale too much. Be careful. Less is more.

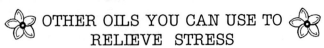

OTHER OILS YOU CAN USE TO RELIEVE STRESS

I have always been sensitive to beauty and great aromas and music and literature. One of my favorite books that I read in my twenties was *Perfume: The Story of a Murderer* by Patrick Suskind. The anti-hero Jean-Baptiste Grenouille has an obsessive pursuit of aromas in his quest to recreate the perfect smell of the ultimate woman. Thank goodness I am not killing anybody to provoke emotions with aromatherapy, like Jean-Baptiste Grenouille was in the novel, but I really do believe that what you smell strongly influences how you feel.

All citrus oils are amazing for helping you decompress smoothly if you are having a Chihuahua-on-the edge moment. In addition to the three oils in ❀ *Pump the Peace*, I also enjoy inhaling any one of these oils straight from the bottle: Basil, Bay laurel, Benzoin, Camphor, Chamomile, Clary Sage (if you do not mind the hay bale smell!), Cedarwood, Coriander, Eucalyptus, Fir, Geranium, Jasmine, Juniper, Lavender, Marjoram, Melissa, Palmarosa, Patchouli, Peppermint, Petitgrain, Ravensara, Pine, Rose, Sage, Sandalwood, Tea tree and Thyme.

Aromatherapy can be used in a variety of ways for many benefits. It is a great solution to help a natural healing process occur. At the end of the book is a simple list of different methods of inhalation and application so you can use essential oils at home or in a massage practice.

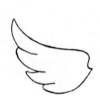

Remember that pain has this most excellent quality. If prolonged it cannot be severe, and if severe it cannot be prolonged.
-Lucius Annaeus Seneca

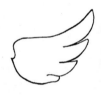

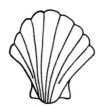

Seashell #2
Welcome Back Your
Healthy Body—Simple Oil
Essentials to Eliminate Pain

Wow, this seashell is one of the highest in demand because so many people are in pain. At least once, almost everyone will suffer from acute or chronic pain. Personally, my pain tolerance is zero. I am not a Rambo. I am more like a Bambi. While working on *Human Target* for 2 seasons, I met Mark, a superhero figure actor who enjoyed doing crazy stunts a lot.

The shooting of the TV series Human Target *was physically demanding along with working long hours. Throughout, Marina was relied on for her restorative shiatsu hands in between scenes. Thanks Marina!*

Mark Valley, Actor

L.A.

No one <u>wants</u> to be in pain, and pain is one of the main

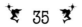

reasons why people book an aromatherapy massage with me. Muscular aches and pains are also the most popular reason to visit the family doctor. This is such a sad reality, and I will do my best to help you feel better.

My aromatherapy clients looking for relief are usually suffering from chronic pain when I first meet them. Usually pain is a combination of physical and mental discomfort. I am in awe of the work of Louise H. Hay, an amazing cancer survivor and metaphysical lecturer who has researched the origins of pain in so many ways. My favorite of her books is ⚝ *You Can Heal Your Life*. She assigns meaning to the different types of pain you can feel in different parts of your body, declaring that these are the physical results of unresolved emotional and spiritual traumas. She offers amazing affirmations to reprogram and jumpstart your healing process. This means you can take charge of your own healing. Brilliant.

With aromatherapy, you have the help of extremely powerful angels called essential oils that can shift you in a very profound way. I believe in miracles. I believe in aromatherapy. When you inhale essential oils, you open the communication between the Source and you. The spirit of the plant becomes available to heal you. The code of healing becomes activated, and the oils, combined with the intention of healing, are mixed with pure love--the highest healing frequency available on the planet (and it is free and unlimited).

Before each session we always set the intention for the client to participate in his or her own healing.

Once they're facedown on the table, I rock my clients gently, asking for permission to work together to relieve the issue. I want you, the client, to focus on the intention of what you want to heal in the session and let go, release it, forgive, or whatever you need to create healing and wholeness.

Sometimes my clients tell me their intention, other times they don't want me to know. Either way, by getting your assent to sign on and participate in your own healing, we double the energy and the power of the massage therapy session.

Some people come to me simply desiring a feeling of relaxation, others are very specific about wanting pain management. Whatever it is, they tell me all the things they want to work on at the beginning.

In my massage sessions, there are many layers of healing happening. A client may go into the frequency they need to relieve the pain, whether they are going back into the energy that created it or are able to create a loving space of surrender.

In the first session, clients usually want to talk a lot. They are afraid, not ready to let go. A lot of times they will say to me afterwards, "I talked too much, I need to talk less next time." I always say, "Good, when you dive into the session, it's definitely going to be more powerful."

I like to let people have their own process and give them options. What they want to do is their decision.

I am very clear with my clients. I tell them, "I'm not here to fix you." The reason I call my pain relief blend "Mr. Fix It" is because it lets me give the power to the oils but also call on the power of great intention to relieve pain.

Also, there is some playfulness in the name. "Mr. Fix It" is somebody who is really good with his hands, a hands-on person. If you're not very good with your hands (or you have pain in hard-to-reach places), you need some extra help. Strong, capable and reliable—that's what "Mr. Fix It" means to me and that's what makes 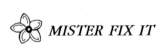 *Mr. Fix It* Essential Oil Blends so effective.

Essential Oils fit very well into the definition of holistic medicine, which treats the patient as a whole, a unified entity. This means treating the wholeness of the body, mind, emotions and spirit. The essential oils are extremely beneficial for activating neurochemicals (serotonin and endorphins, the happy hormones), the signals that communicate from the nervous system to other body systems. When the path is open, you are on the road to healing.

When you come to see me for a session, if your main concern is physical pain or discomfort, we always discuss what happened to cause the injury or pain. The first step is to establish a level of relaxation to help you to cope with the situation. This is where the oils help so beautifully.

I enjoy using essential oils with a massage and clients are also encouraged to bring home a bottle of their beautiful blend to use it on themselves for the next few weeks. For pain management, I have created three blends for the *Mister Fix It* series to support you in your own healing: *Mister Fix It R for Relaxation, Mister Fix It M for Muscles* and *Mister Fix It B for Bones.*

MISTER FIX IT When I was seven years old, I was trying to fly down the stairs at home and I sprained my left ankle. Attempting to conquer my fear of heights, I told myself, "I can do this. I can fly." I also wanted to impress my little sister. Sometimes boys jump off a roof—I tried to fly down the stairs.

In the seventies, physiotherapy and aromatherapy were not

known modalities in my family... Instead, I got some ice on the ankle, and I remember limping like the kangaroo Skippy for many days.

Over the years, I injured this left ankle 15 more times. I had crutches in my apartment always ready and I was using anti-inflammatories for pain. The doctors said, "Your ankle is gone, no more support, no more ligaments."

When I returned from Japan after Shiatsu massage school, I threw my crutches in the garbage. I consciously decided I was not going to sprain my ankle anymore. But it did happen one more time. Looking back, the persistent problem was probably a fear of not having enough support.

The last time I sprained my ankle was in January 2000 in Costa Rica. I had my essential oils with me; I knew what to do. I was able to walk normally and get married the day after.

I was hiking down a mountain after a day of zip-line excitement. I was so proud of myself for conquering my fear of heights. Then I saw a dead poisonous snake. I didn't want to walk over it, so I swerved—but my ankle didn't. I sprawled on the ground in pain.

I was determined to fix this with the oils. A fear came in around the issue of getting married. But instead of cold feet, I got a sprained ankle. Here I had just faced my fear of heights (and I was the only one in the group with no zip-line experience).

I never sprained my ankle ever again afterward. I am probably more confident and grounded than I ever have been when I walk.

So... how did I "Fix It?"

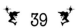

39

Mr. Fix It R BLEND FOR RELAXATION

The first blend I use is R for relaxation, then I apply oils to help to heal the muscle. I like to work in layers. When I sprained my ankle, I used all three *Mr. Fix It* Blends, followed with warm and cold compresses. It's amazing how little scar tissue remains or pain is suffered after a session with me using this method.

I iced the ankle, elevated the leg and applied a blend of Apricot Kernel oil mixed with Basil (*Ocimum basilicum*) for relaxing and calming down the pain in my ankle, Black Pepper (*Piper nigrum*), wonderful for aches and rheumatism as well, Lavender (*Lavendula angustifolia*) for relaxation and inflammation, rheumatism and arthritis, Pine (*Pinus sylvestris*) for muscular aches and pains and rheumatism, and Rosemary (*Rosemarinus officinalis*) for sprains, analgesic for muscular aches and pains as well as rheumatism.

I massaged this blend on my ankle and applied a warm compress for ten minutes, then a cold compress for another ten minutes, which I kept alternating. It was amazing how quickly the stress on my ankle started to melt away. The lymph was working really hard to protect the bone, the ligaments and the muscles. *Mister Fix It R* really helped me to relax and heal.

Mister Fix It M BLEND FOR YOUR MUSCLES

Because I wanted to make sure to be perfectly calm, in the flow and ready for my wedding ceremony on the beach, I applied this second blend on my ankle, *Mister Fix It M* for muscles in need. The Apricot Kernel carrier oil contains these eight essential oils: Clove (*Syzygium aromaticum*), a wonderful analgesic for pain, it numbs the area (remember the dentist?), Eucalyptus (*Eucalyptus globulus*) for aches and pains—also a natural anti-inflammatory, Juniper (*Juniperus communis*), a big help for rheumatism, Marjoram (*Origanum marjorana*) for sprains, bruises, muscular problems, Peppermint (*Mentha piperita*) for inflammation and arthritis and just cooling down the heat, Spearmint (*Mentha spicata*), the little brother of Peppermint that helps with the joy factor, Thyme (*Thymus vulgaris*), great for helping rheumatism, gout, sciatica and muscle pain and spasms, Bulgarian Rose (*Rosa damascena*, AKA *Rose otto*) for muscle spasms and sprains and strains. Again, I massaged this blend on my ankle and applied cold and warm compresses, for ten minutes each.

 ### Mister Fix It B BLEND FOR YOUR BONES

By then, my foot was in great shape! I went to the pool for gentle hydrotherapy with no pressure on the joint and I applied *Mister Fix It B* to make sure my little ankle bones were happy and ready for the big day—my wedding day. This blend is mixed with Apricot Kernel carrier oil with Black Pepper (*Piper nigrum*) for stiffness, sports injuries and broken bones, Camphor (*Cinnamonum camphora*), a very famous ingredient in many muscle pain ointments, great for joints aches and pain and gout, rheumatism and arthritis—the smell is very sharp, Cypress (*Cupressus sempervirens*), quite helpful for reducing swelling, an anti-rheumatic and antispasmodic, Frankincense (*Boswellia carteri*), generally very strong for helping with pain and an anti-inflammatory, Ginger (*Zingiber officinalis*) for swollen joints as well as an analgesic—it also aids in the healing of broken bones, Lavender (*Lavendula angustifolia*) for sports injuries and the calming effect when you have pain, Lemon (*Citrus limonum*) for arthritis and rheumatism and gout, Pine

(*Pinus sylvestris*), excellent if you have pain in your joints and inflammation in your body.

The next day I woke up and my pain was gone. Although a bit stiff, I walked that day and was able to stroll down the aisle (on the beach) to meet my groom. These three ❀ *Mister Fix It R M* & *B* blends saved my wedding day.

I encourage you to either use the essential oil that you like the most as a single oil in your favorite method of application, or, if you are in need of the ultimate power of more essential oils, just use these three blends.

I first met Marina 10 years ago. At that time I had been seeing many different massage therapists to try and alleviate that extreme pain that I feel in my right arm and hand, but I never came out of my session feeling any better...until I came into contact with the beautiful hands of Marina and her aromatherapy! The way she puts her whole body and soul into the work that she does is amazing. You feel her loving energy in every touch. Just after one session I began to feel my pain dissipate and have continued to enjoy her touch ever since. She is my angel of massage :) Using the **Mister Fix it** *blend daily on my right forearm has improved my mobility tremendously.*

Sabina Gallant

Vancouver, B.C.

MY STONE HELPERS

I have met so many wonderful people in these last few years of my life in Vancouver, my precious clients. I do not feel that I have a job; it is more of a passion. My hands are my best friends, my sisters of light. They guide me and know what to do. I also love using jade stones during my sessions. Did you know that nephrite jade is the official provincial gemstone of British Columbia? This stone is superb for holding the heat and helping you dissolve stress and anxiety.

I also use river stones to help your energy speed up and to activate your joy factor, and black volcanic stones that allow you to let go of sadness and nostalgia. These stones help you ground yourself as well. I am also very fond of promoting the release of any pain and aches and discomfort with the help of hydrotherapy.

 ## THE SOAKING SOLUTION

When I lived in Montreal, in my twenties, I discovered a great hydrotherapy center called Ovarium. You could soak inside a big floating tank full of two thousand cups of Epsom salt and Dead Sea salt mixed with warm water, with your ears immersed underwater. Gregorian chants played while you relaxed in the water. Divine. This was so soothing for me in my twenties; it helped me to relieve a lot of stress. It is also, it turns out, the fastest way to open your third eye to help unleash your intuition.

This place was packed with people looking to calm down, relax, reduce pain and receive insights for creativity. I saw many artists there, students like me looking for a boost of endorphins to be able to focus and deliver brilliant exams, lawyers before a big court case, future mothers wanting to get really focused and grounded before their delivery date, and older people with physical pain.

The session was one hour long and you would receive the loving care of all these salts helping your body to let go of lactic acid build-up caused by stress and pain. I wish I could have this big egg of water in my living room! I am a mermaid, I love my water, I love bathing!

When my clients leave my caring hands, I ask them to have a bath after the massage to help release lactic acid, and to use essential oils in the bath. Clients who don't follow up with a bath sometimes have more pain because of the residual acid from the tension points that were massaged and released. Without a bath, these discomforts could last up to a few days after the session.

To get rid of acidity and the rest of the toxins, you need only to spend 20 minutes. Go to the health food store and buy sea salt—sea salt from the Dead Sea is the ultimate treat—it is loaded with minerals. If you journey to the Dead Sea, you can float easily on the water because of the high mineral content. Epsom salts will also do the trick.

When you have discomfort, just reach for your favorite oil discussed in this chapter and mix eight drops of it in one cup of Dead Sea salt or Epsom salt and pour it in your bath. The osmosis will happen in 20 minutes of soaking. It's so easy to let go of the discomfort with aromatherapy and salt.

Aromatherapy used in combination with stone therapy and hydrotherapy is super fireworks powerful!

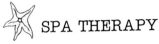 SPA THERAPY

Back east, my sisters and family are the creators of Spa Natureau in Mandeville, in the lower Laurentian mountains of Quebec. This is one of the best-kept secrets for hydrotherapy centers in the province of Quebec. They even have an aromatherapy room with a great diffuser featuring different essential oils for the day. Your body and soul will travel in pure bliss. You can soak in these baths to help your skin to cleanse, your circulation to improve, and you will feel energized and relaxed at the same time. For more information, visit www. spanatureau.com.

Because I live on the west coast of Canada, I go to Scandinave Spa in Whistler. I love to soak in this outdoor spa in the mountains and forest. I stay there for the whole day and relax in the eucalyptus steam bath or the wood-burning Finnish sauna to stimulate blood circulation and release toxins. Then I plunge into the Nordic waterfall or cold shower to close the pores and strengthen my immune system. Their basins are filled with mineral waters. I love lounging in their solariums or hammocks to allow my cardiovascular system to regulate itself and my blood circulation to decrease.

HOW TO KEEP THE JUST-MASSAGED FEELING GOING . . .

Physical pain is one thing but emotional pain is also important to heal. Are you in emotional or mental pain right now? Are you shy, insecure, sad or even lost sometimes? When I am feeling low I really need courage, focus, love, and a pat on my shoulders to get going. That is why I enjoy the support of essential oils on the go. Your nose knows, and when you inhale the oils, you get and instant boost of natural stimulation.

My *Nose Job* inhalers are made just for you to pick yourself up when you are down or tired and to stave off physical pain. I believe pure potential is limitless. Open up and receive the help of the essential oils so you can live in your frontal lobe and stay in the moment. When your hypothalamus gland, pineal gland and third eye are wide open and vibrating full force, you will manifest miracles. To learn more on this topic, look into Kadea Metara, an amazing healer who prepared me very well since 2001 to accept my gifts and start to share with this book. Her website is www.kadea.org.

As I mentioned, I enjoy working and playing with the angel cards of Doreen Virtue for guidance with the archangels. Michael, Raphael, Chamuel, Jophiel, Haniel, Gabriel, Sandalphon and Metatron and many more are in my daily life. I took Doreen's class in Vancouver years ago and I got my huge heart-shaped rock of Amethyst "wings" necklace from her. Archangel Michael is certainly one of my favorite guardians. I usually wear this necklace when I am playing with essential oils. It feels so good to combine the crystals with the oils and the love intention. I also attended an amazing spiritual retreat in Arizona at Miraval Resort recently, where I connected deeply with special people in the intuitive healing world. Doreen is a fantastic clairvoyant and metaphysical leader and she helped us to open up to our sacred blessings with so much respect and love with the support of the angels. We are the Equinox Circle. We love you, Doreen! Find out more at ✩ www.angeltherapy. com.

A part of my life mission is to help people to elevate their life force naturally with the help of essential oils. Cancer care is a very important goal as well as helping to introduce essential oils in hospitals. I want to ignite inspiration into the hearts of young people to use essential oils to boost their energy and health naturally. The use of ❀ *Nose Job* inhalers is part of the plan. I would like to start teaching young students to use the oils for opening their vortex of creativity. The inhalers are going to help them to stay focused, strong, courageous, happy and inspired. When I am studying, I use ❀ *Nose Job Crystal Clear* to keep airways open, ❀ *Nose Job Sports* to retain my mental focus, ❀ *Nose Job I Believe* to elevate my confidence when I talk in front of a group, *Nose Job Pure Potential* to open up my vortex of creativity and *Nose Job Limitless* to ground myself in my peaceful warrior energy. These inhalers are proprietary formulas.

Magical Marina's Massage
Felt like a "Fairy on a Leaf."

Renee Strong

B.C. Canada

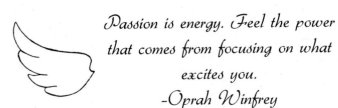 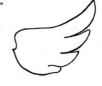

Passion is energy. Feel the power
that comes from focusing on what
excites you.
-Oprah Winfrey

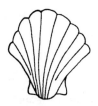

Seashell #3
Aromatherapy Secrets to Increase Your Vibration and Amplify Your Energy

What is energy? Everything has a unique frequency. Good energy, bad energy, good vibes, bad vibes, high energy, low energy. I am fascinated by energy and frequency levels. A long time ago I read the book  *The Cure for all Diseases* by Hulda Regehr Clark, Ph.D.,N.D. She stated "The human body broadcasts electrically, just like a radio station, but over a wide band of frequencies and very low voltages, which is why it has not been detected and measured until now."

She discovered that every living organism has a frequency and a bandwidth. For insects this is between 1,000,000 Hz and 1,500,000 Hz. Cockroaches were the highest amongst insects she tested. No wonder you always see them surviving in apocalyptic movie scenarios.

People with the highest frequency don't get sick; they have good immune systems. People with low immune systems vibrate at lower frequencies.

After you drink alcohol, your frequency will be lower for the next few hours. If you start feeling bad, it's wise to avoid alcohol, sugar and processed food. Drink some good herbal tea to flush your system and your frequency will go up.

Do you know how many muscles we need to smile? 17.

Do you know how many muscles we need to frown? 47.

Let's conserve energy and <u>smile</u>. If you are happy, please tell your face. I was raised by a mother who always said that a smile is the key to attracting what you want in life. My mother is a very good people person when it comes to finding solutions to their problems. When we had the family business, she gave clients service to the max. A client would come to buy the newspaper and would leave with a whole grocery bag. "Oh do you need this? If you are buying that, you will surely need this." My mother has an eye for detail and a smile that is always at attention.

That is a big reason why my pet peeve is people who have a <u>concrete face</u>. I admit I have an issue with that! Drop the stone cold face and put on a smile and your life will smile back at you. When your vibrations are high and joyful, have you noticed how life is flowing and people just think that you are a lollipop and sweet as bubble gum? They just want to be in your bubble because they feel great around your energy. The power of a genuine smile is certainly the key to positive vibrations. "Smile and you shall receive" is my motto. It's hard to smile and then try to stay angry or down. The energy we have as human beings is our gift to share.

What is your gift? What are you bringing to the table? Are you conscious of your energy level? Because we are like walking antennas, we are always emitting and receiving waves of frequency. When I am not feeling so good and I am worried about something or I'm angry, I feel a huge black cloud over my head following me everywhere I go until I switch my vibrations from negative to positive. That is the time I get my spritzer out and spritz myself with essential oils. It really helps to get rid of this dark vortex or heavy umbrella over my head. I really recommend citrus essential oils for that. The blend for this energy seashell is called ✿ *Pump the Joy*.

I always want to be in high-energy mode. That is why I am highly addicted to essential oils. I know now that they are the fastest ticket for me to switch my mood. When I am vibrating at a high level, I feel like the sky is the limit. Energy is a great fuel when it is elevated, catalyzed, focused, respected and cherished. I always tell my clients that I am high on essential oils and I rarely get sick because of it. I have touched a lot of people in my life. I started seriously studying massage techniques when I turned 18 years old. I have spent 27 years of doing massages here and there, as well as seriously massaging 500 people per year in the last 15 years, and I am still standing! I have performed over 10,000 massages so far. Wow!

I rarely get sick and I know that the oils are my Soldiers of Love. Love is, by the way, the ultimate highest frequency for healing. The oils, combined with the intention of making you feel higher, is my ultimate goal and focus in life. I really believe that, like the physicist Dr. William Tiller predicted, "Future medicine will be based on controlling energy frequencies in the body." Read more about Dr. Tiller at www.heartmath.com.

I really admire the book ✕ *The Healing Code* by Alexander Loyd, which contains a great deal of precious information on how to heal yourself by neutralizing a negative frequency thought with a positive truth focus statement. Instead of saying, "I don't want to be sick," you say, "I am vibrating with excellent health right now." I really believe that when you are able to discover the thoughts and emotions that are stopping you from receiving what you want, you can move and manifest very quickly. If you switch your negative state to positive bliss by awareness and intention with a love vibration and essential oils, your life will transform profoundly.

Essential oils have frequencies. Different essential oils have different frequencies, a subtle buzz created by their bio-electric property. I have also seen pictures of light (like the aura) of the essential oil. There are still a lot of unanswered questions regarding the exact level of megahertz, but it has been said that when you are using Rose essential oil you connect with 320 megahertz.

Many varied university researchers have also found that when you are sick with cancer you usually vibrate under 42 megahertz, and if you are healthy, you vibrate at 75 megahertz and more. If you have psychic abilities you are able to vibrate at more then 200 megahertz. I can't tell you for sure that this information is the truth, but I feel that when I am full of love and life and good intention I feel <u>fantastic</u>! When your energy is high, you cannot be sick. Elevation of your frequencies is definitely the goal for us to stay healthy. When I get stuck in the mind, I get stressed and overwhelmed. But when I'm in high vibration mode I can move mountains. When I use a lot of oils, my vibration is usually very high.

Everybody is looking for ways to get energy nowadays— yoga, extreme sports, energy drinks, oxygen bars, runner's high… because what happens when your energy is low? When you have been running on empty and feeling negative energy for too long, there is a good chance you are getting bombarded with negative frequencies.

Depression is a big problem right now in our over-stimulated society. The Mayo Clinic reports say that depression is a serious illness that causes changes in mood, thinking, physical wellbeing and behavior. It can affect all aspects of a person's life. Depression is caused by a complex set of physical, psychological and environmental factors. Sometimes a stressful life event can trigger depression. In other cases, depression seems to occur spontaneously with no identifiable cause. No matter what triggers it, depression is much more than grieving or a bout of the blues.

Depression may occur only once in a person's life. Often, however, it occurs repeatedly with depression-free periods in between. It also may be an ongoing condition, requiring treatment over a lifetime. Depression affects 18 million Americans. According to Health Canada and Statistics Canada, in any given year, about 7%, between 13 million and 14 million people will experience a depressive disorder.

Aromatherapy is a complementary health modality. The safe use of essential oils within the practice of holistic aromatherapy can help enhance your overall emotional outlook and can be used to accompany other traditional and alternative modalities that combat depression. Over the last ten years I have noticed a big resurgence of antidepressant users. My goal is to make sure the client on antidepressants starts to feel better, more relaxed and empowered with the essential oils they use after their sessions with me.

I've seen enormous changes in clients who have had depression and consistently come to me for aromatherapy massage. Once they are able to go off antidepressants, they start going to the gym, changing jobs, changing relationships. The people who stick to antidepressants are too stressed out to make changes.

While working in the film industry, I saw so many women using Ativan, Prozac, Valium and Zoloft. Starting in their thirties, with the long hours on set, they would pop an Ativan before bed, then use wake-up pills and drink several coffees throughout the day. They all looked older than their biological age!

Since I started working in the film industry as a stand-in and massaging the crew and actors, I have been able to educate them about healthy alternatives. Now many of these same women who were depressed and popping pills are using essential oil diffusers in the makeup trailer. Professional makeup artists and hairdressers are now creating this pleasant, healthy, delicious atmosphere that is elevating everyone's mood.

These "drama queen trailers" can create a toxic atmosphere to work in if you don't have a good team. Working with lead actors force many of the crew to give massages—massaging egos! I would ignore their egos and massage their shoulders using the oils. Instead of killing each other, everybody in the trailer got "high" off the oils. Of course, the negative people would hate me, but I felt happy so I didn't care!

What do you do if you're a hair or makeup person? The actor sits in the chair for a long time. You have to talk to the star and listen to their stories and complaints. So the artists would hire me for a spot on the weekend, and tell their actors, "Oh you *have* to see Marina!" I would calm them down so the actor was easier to work with come Monday morning.

I would call it the "Sedation Syndrome" and work on actors, actresses—even their dogs! They called me "Marina the Cleaner." I always liked it when I could get one-on-one with them; I'm really good at shifting their energy, and the makeup team would be grateful. They'd come back to work on Monday to find the actors' attitudes in check. I am so glad that Tone, a former make-up artist, used the aromatherapy to handle the stress and long hours on movie sets.

When I met Marina "Mermaid," she had a small mobile service traveling from movie sets to movie sets in Vancouver, "rescuing" actors and film crews in their high stress careers. I was a make-up artist at the time and became addicted to escaping into the world of Marina's aromatherapy massages. She and her sessions were a haven of relaxation and calmness much needed in my line of work. I always left with newfound energy and positivity, ready to take on the world. "Marina Mermaid" products followed me everywhere and I still use them today! I thank her for being the "beginning" of my journey towards self-realization.

I eventually took the leap, quit the film industry and returned to Europe. This gave me a chance to share precious time with my family and the opportunity to make peace with my dear father before he passed away too quickly from cancer. My new life attracted my soulmate and our two amazing boys shortly after. Apart from being co-owners and business partners we also shared the love of France and built our dream home there. I am honored and thankful for still having Marina in my life. She has been a true friend, a healing angel and a catalyst for change in my life for many years. I am so very happy that she takes the time to travel to France where she blesses our family and the French community here with her amazing aromatherapy sessions. This book is her official launch as a new ambassador for Essential oils.

I wish you all the success and happiness life has to offer Marina! Merci mon amie…

Tone Rorvik

Le Petit Bardeche, www.holidaycottagesandvillas.com

France

Mary Steenburgen and Ted Danson once hired me to massage the whole crew when they were shooting the miniseries *Talking to Heaven* by James Van Praagh.

They had heard about me and I massaged them with a chair massage, which they loved. It was very smart of them to do this for the crew. Everybody got high on the oils and it was a calm and joyful set. Some producers buy $500 worth of coffee for the crew. This makes everyone more acidic and more stressed out than ever.

Movie sets can be an incredibly stressful atmosphere. Because of the expense of making a film, every second the clock is ticking costs money, so people are on edge. They work long hours for months at a time and actors go in early for makeup and can sometimes stay very late at night (which is not good for their hormonal system and cortisol levels). Crew members are often sleep-deprived, and not exercising or eating right, which only adds to the stress in their bodies. Inhaling essential oils creates a more alkaline atmosphere, happier and attuned to the vibration of love.

Hilary Swank also paid for the entire crew to enjoy chair massages; she is an advocate of holistic medicine. And I gave Brooke Shields special bath products for her to enjoy at night in her hotel. I get shy when I do this. Sometimes I give them a little gift and then run away! Brooke talks to everybody, is polite and funny and likes to knit on set.

As for me, I have this gift. I have the energy and willpower to sustain these crazy hours. I can go for months, then when the shoot is over, I refocus and regroup. I am a Fire Horse, after all!

Being in the flow is my favorite way to be. When we live in

the present, life is so much better. Sometimes I get carried away by the mad hamster or possessed Chihuahua of my mental chatter we talked about in the Stress Seashell. However, once I notice his presence, I tell him thanks for sharing and then spritz myself with ❀ *Pump the Joy* blend.

Knowledge is great, but when you take action, you open the gates of flowing energy. Take action now in your own healing and notice if you are transforming your energy to be in the flow.

Do you feel tired all the time? If your thyroid gland is sluggish and "hypo," you are probably exhausted when you wake up. This master gland is the queen of your metabolism and it is very important to get it activated to improve your health and vitality. Since you are on a jumpstarting the metabolism program, book yourself for a full general exam with your doctor and ask to receive your full blood test panel for your TSH.

Sometimes you have to pay to get this information. You need this. Remember, you are building the file of your wellness freedom, all your medical tests belong to you as well. If you live in Canada, register on <u>www.ehealth.ca</u> to receive a copy of your blood test results. You can study these with your health professional. Information is <u>power</u>.

Now, how to jumpstart your metabolism? For me, it starts with a massive eight hours of sleep. For some people even eight hours is not enough. The timeframe to get the best quality sleep is very crucial. That is when your hormonal system is at its peak ability to rebuild and recharge. I enjoy being in bed by 10:00 pm and waking up by 7:00 am. If I do not get enough sleep, I am grumpy, moody and sensitive. I need my sleep!

Cortisol is one of many hormones that our body creates. It is also one of the major hormones that controls our ability to lose or gain fat and energy.

We all need a certain amount of cortisol in our body because that's what wakes us up in the morning, but too much of it promotes fat storage and what I call blah-ness (feeling lethargic and unenthusiastic). Cortisol is activated by two occurrences: daylight intake and stress. Stress could be caused by physical and mental factors as well as pollutants (what we ingest and absorb from the environment). Regarding daylight, the body is very intelligent, but it cannot tell the difference between daylight and the light from computers and televisions.

That kernel of information actually makes it feasible to control a large part of our daily stress. Keep in mind that our bodies have a natural cortisol pattern. It has been found that cortisol peaks in the morning. The levels start rising drastically from 5:30 am or so with the sunrise, until 9:30 in the morning. So, it makes sense that controlling the amount of simulated daylight, computer and TV light at night would reduce the production of cortisol quite a bit. Not to mention the break that your adrenal glands will get (that is where all hormones are made).

Now, speaking of the adrenal glands, they produce most, if not all, of your hormones like your testosterone, estrogen, DHEA (the youth hormone) and yes, the infamous cortisol. The adrenal glands only have so much juice to create all of these hormones, but cortisol takes priority over the others.

You see, your body only wants to protect itself. If you give it the message you need cortisol by giving it daylight from your TV and computer late at night, there is only so much juice available to produce the other hormones. You then get what is called "cortisol steal." Your adrenals will give your body what it needs for survival and will take from Peter to give to Paul—and that leads to hormonal imbalance. Yes, you can go to your doctor and get on a hormonal balancing program by prescription. But wouldn't it be much easier to do it right the first time around by controlling stress levels and late night light absorption from the get-go? For more information please register to www.agilispeed.com to receive "The Missing Piece" Special Report.

I have also invested in the best sleep system ever: the foam memory system Tempur-Pedic® is fantastic. It is so easy to jumpstart your energy level when you are rested, it makes you feel that anything is possible. Also when you go to bed, make sure your room is dark with an effective light-blocking window treatment.

During the day you can keep your blood sugar stable by eating snacks, so your body will feel nourished and loved instead of experiencing fatigue, hunger, even headaches. At night, your body also needs the comfort of knowing what to expect. Give your body a routine; try to go to bed at the same time every night.

Imagine turning off the TV or computer at 8 pm, dimming the lights and getting ready for bed, then enjoying a good book or magazine on your comfortable mattress until sleep time. It's a relaxing way to wind down and show your body and your hormones some love. Diffusing essential oils before you go to bed makes it even more pleasurable. Or spritz **Pump the Joy** or single oils Jasmine, soothing Neroli or the flower with the highest frequency, Rose oil, on your sheets to enjoy their calming and uplifting fragrance all night long.

I have made balancing and uplifting your stressed-out

system simple with three easy spritzers. In a massage session with clients, I use the traditional healing oils, then I spritz *Pump the Joy* over their heads to bring them to an even higher frequency.

To close the session and clear the space, I call the names of the oils, and strike my chime eight times with infinity signs to make sure any negative energy is gone from their body, me or the healing room.

If they like, they can purchase blends to take home with them to put in their baths with sea salt to purify, dispel negativity and alleviate stress, tiredness and depression. I do recommend a bath after a massage to prevent soreness and allow the body to detox. Everyone has different ailments, so I promote different oils or blends in spritzer form as well. Spritzers are so great; they're easy to use and portable. There is no dripping or spillage of oils on clothes or sheets, just a cool, refreshing spray.

Many high-powered women come to see me because they know taking the time to de-stress is part of their success. Relaxing and turning their brain off for a bit also opens the window to ideas, creativity and intuition. Many of my clients make more money than their husbands—30% of women make more than their spouses in Canada.

Hmm… maybe I need to make $ "Pump the Dough" $ to spritz on their husbands…

 Pump the Joy: Blend for alleviating depression, adrenal fatigue and low thyroid function.

Single oils include:

Peppermint. Top note, uplifting. Botanical name: *Mentha piperita*.

Safety data: Non-toxic, non-irritant, but possible sensitization due to menthol. Not to be used if you are pregnant and also breastfeeding. Use in moderation, not compatible with homeopathic treatment.

Peppermint is great for mental fatigue.

In ❀ *Pump the Joy*, the Peppermint oil is used in a very low concentration just for the "aoumfff" sparks for freshness.

Bergamot. Top note, antidepressant. Botanical name: *Citrus bergamia.*

Safety data: Make sure that your Bergamot is a bergapten-free oil because bergapten (also known as furocoumarins) is the chemical in bergamot that causes phototoxicity (skin irritation after sunlight exposure).

Bergamot oil was first sold in the Italian city named Bergamot in Lombardy. The oil has been used in Italian folk medicine for many years. It is very powerful for stress-related conditions and depression and it has a refreshing and uplifting quality. Did you know that Bergamot is the flavoring in Earl Grey tea?

Neroli (orange blossom). Base note, super antidepressant. Botanical name: *Citrus aurantium var. amara.*

Safety data: Super safe! Non-toxic, non-irritant, non-sensitizing, non-phototoxic.

Once upon a time there was an Italian princess named Nerola. Because she loved wearing orange blossoms as a perfume, it came to be known as Neroli. The essential oil pressed from the delicate white flowers is very expensive but super fabulous. This "ninja mood enhancer" of essential oils makes you feel uplifted big time. I use it a lot to help brides calm down before the wedding ceremony. Neroli body treatments are so amazing. Very good for highly emotional states, depression and nervousness.

Jasmine. Base note, uplifting. Botanical name: *Jasminum officinale.*

Safety data: Non-toxic, non-irritant, generally non-sensitizing, but some individuals could have an allergic reaction. Not to be used if pregnant.

Jasmine is a wonderful oil to help to let go of raw frustration. The jasmine sambac dried flowers are also used for jasmine tea. If you are a giver, this is your ticket for replenishment of the heart. Jasmine is the warrior oil when you are down and burned out and at the end of your rope. It will propel you back to nirvana. Also, Jasmine is a powerful aphrodisiac and in his book ✻ *Aromatherapy Workbook*, Marcel Lavabre describes that when Cleopatra used to sail to greet the Roman Emperor Marc Anthony, the sails of her ship were soaked in jasmine, one of the most aphrodisiac fragrances. Marc Anthony fell so deeply in love with Cleopatra that he gave up his empire to follow her.

Rose. Botanical name: *Rosa damascena* (rose otto) and *Rosa centifolia* (rose maroc).

Safety data: Non-toxic, non-irritant, non-sensitizing, but not to be used with children, also use caution during pregnancy.

Rose oil is fabulous for depression. It is one of the most expensive oils in the world. The healing properties of the rose have been utilized in medicine (*materia medica*) throughout the ages. In his classic book ✻ *The Art of Aromatherapy*, written in 1977, Robert B. Tisserand says that the rose is expensive because rose petals contain very little essence, and up to 2,000 kg of petals maybe needed to produce I kg of oil. My Rose oil is diluted, which makes it affordable. Some Rose oils are in the $300 and $400 range for a 10 ml bottle, and some cost even more than that.

Rose essential oil is used as the symbol of the soul, love and purity. It has been dedicated to Aphrodite, the Greek goddess of sexual love and beauty, and her Roman equivalent, Venus. Because the scent of Rose is so sensual, the Romans scattered rose petals on the bridal beds for wedding nights... a tradition now replaced by throwing confetti. History shows us that the Egyptian rose was the one Cleopatra used to seduce Mark Anthony. She was fond of rose petals and hydrosols and oils. Athenaeus, a writer of the times, records that Cleopatra covered the floors of her palace with fresh rose petals to a depth of half a meter. The sails of her royal barge were drenched in rosewater when sailing to meet Julius Caesar. Definitely one of her trademarks! Also in her bedroom surrounding the bed, she and her lover walked through a thick sultry layer of rose petals as deep as autumn leaves.

I often wonder how I would have enjoyed being incarnated in the body of Nefertiti or Cleopatra. Cleopatra was a goddess of sensuality, loving to soak in baths with milk, herbs, essential oils and flower petals. These rituals with these gifts of nature kept her young and powerful. She was a very good businesswoman and she knew how to use nature to elevate her vibrations.

Once again for this precious blend we are keeping the life force of the essential oils in a fresh jojoba carrier oil. Jojoba is highly penetrative and very stable. It does not go rancid and has no contraindications.

Rose Hydrosol (floral water left after distillation of the roses for oil) is a more affordable way to enjoy this oil in a spritzer form. Rose is considered the highest frequency flower, so many spiritual people use roses or the image of roses to clean their own energy or the energy of their clients. I use the image of a necklace of roses around my crown for protection and cleansing my energy before, during and after a session. Using rose spray in your home, spritzing it on yourself and your loved ones is an excellent way to maintain high vibrations for everyone you love.

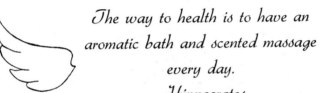

The way to health is to have an aromatic bath and scented massage every day.
-Hippocrates

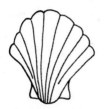

Seashell #4

Diminish Cellulite and Puffiness—Increase Circulation on the Inside So You Can Flow with Life on the Outside

This seashell is one of my favorites. Why? Because we all want to have a good circulation and a strong lymphatic system in order to stay lean and energetic and healthy. Are you suffering from puffy ankles that feel like watermelons? Puffy hands and feet as well? You should know that if your blood circulation is in top shape, your lymphatic system is also happy. If not, then you have to deal with puffiness, sluggishness, varicose veins, tiredness, cellulite, fat cell augmentation, skin issues, and feelings of sickness because you are too toxic. There is so much you can naturally do to regain vibrant flowing circulation and a healthy lymphatic system.

I used to be almost 200 pounds when I was a teenager. I would eat so much of the wrong food and I really never exercised then. I had to make a conscious decision about how I was going to live my life. At that time I was enjoying food to excess, getting puffier and puffier, and I had to force myself to exercise. My clothes were not fitting and my family was telling me I looked rounder. I learned that circulation and lymphatic systems needed to be honored so I could have the energy to do what I wanted to do in my life.

I always had very low blood pressure and I was partying a lot, drinking alcohol and smoking cigarettes in my twenties. I could be really fat, then, a few months later, super lean, trying different diets to reach balance in my weight. Now in my forties, I feel healthier than <u>ever</u>. Here are my secrets to improve your circulation and lymphatic flow.

In Latin, *Lympha* means clear water. First of all, our lymphatic system is like a beautiful garbage removal system. But because it is totally dependent on the quality of your circulatory system, it needs extra help to do its job. The lymph has no pump and depends on muscular compression and body movement to move the fluids in your body. Breathing consciously, stretching, doing yoga, making love and exercising will activate your circulatory system and boost your lymph.

LIBERTY WITH THE OILS

I did a lymph pump foot massage for five minutes on a client in a wheelchair and she felt so much more revived, plus her feet were not cold anymore. I used a bit of this lymph decongestant: pine essential oil (*Pinus sylvestris*) in my hands before I gave her the lymph pump and the giggle-giggle ankle shake. I also massaged a beautiful 17-year-old paraplegic and her legs and ankles and feet were so much warmer after the aromatherapy massage. She had a big smile on her face, and said she could feel electricity in her toes, and that made her happy.

I gave her a beautiful olfactory rainbow trip where she inhaled different oils in my hands cupped over her nose. The limbic system will set you free, giving you a ticket to travel in your imagination and create the life you desire. It opens up your frontal lobe where the intuition and the love frequency live. Activating the limbic system helps you live in the present and essential oils can connect you with your higher self to bring more peace into your life. Just look at the way most people close their eyes when they smell the oils, going into that deep and loving space. The lower rear part of the brain is activated by fear. The oils keep you in the gentle, active, expansive section of the brain. Just as reactivating a memory of a former triumph can help an athlete succeed in a game, scents can also connect you with emotionally loving moments so you can carry that frequency forward anytime you desire.

The female energy knows how to access and maximize this pure bliss. This means liberty with the essential oils. It is the yin instinct. It has been my experience that women are attracted to essential oils more often than men. They are more open to trying them. Please make sure you open the senses of any friends or family members who are living with paralysis or in a wheelchair. God bless them for showing us to be grateful for our health.

I learned from Anthony Robbins' programs and Peak Potentials (T. Harv Eker) wellness seminars that jumping on a mini trampoline ten minutes a day was the best way to give yourself a mini lymphatic drainage. How cool is that? My best friend, a hypnotherapist and holistic guru named Eric did ten minutes of rebounding per day on his mini trampoline with his favorite therapist, Mister Magoo, his 18-year-old cat. Super cool.

Oh and by the way, what's up with essential oils and cats? Cats are very curious by nature. While they are attracted by the aromas, please do not attempt to massage them with essential oils and always let them come to you first if they want to inhale essential oils from the bottle. I have seen a lot of cats wanting to be touched and massaged with essential oils but I am cautious and only let them smell from the bottle.

I believe in pet therapy and Dr. Erika Friedmann of Brooklyn College found that pet owners have healthier hearts than heart attack patients who don't have a dog, cat or other pets. In her studies reported in *The American Journal of Cardiology* in 2003, she found that pet owners have shorter hospital stays, few doctor visits, take less medication for high blood pressure and cholesterol, and don't have as much trouble falling asleep at night. Pet therapy will help you to lower your stress level, lower your blood pressure and elevate your happy hormones levels of dopamine, oxytocin and endorphins.

Exercising is mega important and body scrubbing is also a very smart way to move your lymph and your circulation. Your skin will be smooth as a peach too.

BODY SCRUBBING WITH ✗ Renaissance Glove, ⚜ Mermaid Soaps AND ❀ ESSENTIAL OIL BLENDS

I have been showing my clients how to perform body scrubbing on a regular basis to improve their circulation. You can start with dry brushing to remove the dead cells and improve the cleansing ability of your bloodstream. This dry exfoliation should take you a good eight minutes to perform before you get in the shower. Your skin is your largest organ. When the skin is clean and scrubbed, the circulation is so much better. It is a purification ritual that you owe to yourself. I like to perform dry brushing exfoliation once a week, and use the glove wet the other six days.

THE RENAISSANCE GLOVE

The best glove on the market that I have found is the **Renaissance Glove** by Daniele Henkel in Montreal, Quebec. This glove helps to loosen ingrown hair and contributes to the body's beauty and health, all while conveying a marvelous feeling of wellbeing and relaxation. I describe it as "the tongue of a cat licking you." I kid you not, wait till you try it. It is made of 100% Viscose, a hypoallergenic material that is easy to dry and easy to take care of. It is like your new pet. You will <u>love it unconditionally</u>.

I also just adore the feeling of waking up in the morning with a gentle Renaissance brushing and showering with my own aromatherapy soap line that is paraben-free with no propylene glycol. I had to start making my own line because I have a lot of cancer survivors in my clientele, and they are very aware of the chemical overload in our world.

Also, I am an Aries Fire Horse, and need lots of water to balance my hot fire. Hydrotherapy is my sacred time when I receive insights for my creations to express my artistic side. When I am playing in water or soaking in mineral waters (Scandinave Spa in Whistler or at my sisters' Spa Natureau in Quebec), I imagine the water purifying my body and washing away my fears. It is magic. If I have a question, I take a shower or an aromatherapy bath to receive the best guidance. Thank God for my Renaissance scrubbing sessions.

RENAISSANCE SCRUBBING

I have been practicing this natural cleansing for years—it is the best lymphatic boost for me. Always move the toxins out toward the heart. I brush myself, first of all, from the ankle, calf, thigh, and buttocks in circular movements toward the heart and then I brush my abdomen in a clockwise motion. I then start again on my wrists and arms and put them up in the air and move toward the armpit to make sure the toxins are flowing in the right direction back to the thoracic ducts (your highway for the lymph) under each clavicle. I then start brushing gently on the sternum and massage each breast so they too will drain in the armpits. This is very good for your breasts as well.

Your lymph flows throughout your body, and in some areas it is more concentrated: in the groin area; under the armpits; an inch bellow the belly button for the descending colon and the reproductive system; down the front of the chest, sternum and along the outer sides of the neck and jawbone. This technique is very invigorating and I prefer to use my own gel soaps to get the essential oils into my body every day.

When people come to see me and they are exhausted, stressed or in pain, acting lethargic and sluggish, they usually are too toxic and have lots of dead skin. Their skin just falls off as I massage them. I tell them they need to scrub because their skin is not able to excrete the toxins. Then I send them home with a **Renaissance Glove** and they say, "Thank you so much, I feel better, my skin is healthy and so smooth!"

Here are some of my gel body soaps. They make great hand soaps as well.

MARINA MERMAID BODY GEL SOAP KIT

The *Creamsicle Citrus Splash* contains Vanilla, Sweet Orange, Lemon, Grapefruit and Lime in a base of castile soap with saponified organic coconut oil, olive oil, castor oil, jojoba oil, glycerin and vitamin E. Afterwards I like to anoint my whole body with my different body lotions.

I find that guys really dig my ✺ *Gladiator Awakening* body gel as much as girls, because it wakes you up quickly. It is the same soap base with Peppermint (*Mentha piperita*) and Spearmint (*Mentha Spicata*). It's perfect if you are a gladiator— you will be the winner of the combat if you have a big day ahead of you.

✺ *Lavender de France* body gel is a classic gel soap to use, especially at night when you want to calm down. It's also wonderfully atmospheric for an evening bath. My clients tell me their bathroom smells like Provence. They want to smell it all the time, so they also use it as a hand soap.

✺ *After Sex Glow* body gel soap helps you maintain your ultimate smiley face after good "connecting" sessions... this is a luxurious gel soap for when you want to elevate your natural pheromones and sexual energy before a date, or just maintain a sweet sexy attractive smell for pleasuring yourself. Rrrrr. Ylang Ylang (*Cananga odorata*) is the magic aphrodisiac essential oil in this sexy soap.

✺ *Buddha Yoga Fresh* body gel soap is great before your yoga or meditation class. Containing Lemongrass (*Cymbopogon*), this soap will help purify your skin and bloodstream and is amazing for cellulite control. This is an excellent essential oil for purification that I enjoy using in honor of the goddess White Tara to cleanse the inner self.

I like to use natural body lotions as well so I feel hydrated, with smooth, soft skin all day. Here are my body lotions:

✺ 73 ✺

MARINA MERMAID BODY LOTION KIT

Creamsicle Body Lotion contains plenty of Vanilla and Mandarin essential oils.

Marie-Jeanne de France Lotion with French Lavender, to honor my dear friend and mentor, the founder of a very successful cosmetic business in France. *Je t'aime.*

Aloha Mermaid Lotion with fresh sacred Kukui oil from Hawaii, Plumeria and Gardenia flower essences. Each time I inhale it, it brings me back to the Island of Maui, one of my favorite obsessions.

After Sex Glow Body Lotion to honor the hotness of our sensuality with the aphrodisiac Ylang Ylang. Sweet and sexy, it's great for a man or woman.

Buddha Yoga Fresh Body Lotion to purify your Namaste ritual with Lemongrass essential oil and keep you crispy clean and well hydrated.

Gladiator Awakening Body Lotion to keep your skin fresh with Peppermint and Spearmint essential oils.

All these body lotions are made with <u>love</u>, aqua, organic shea butter, mango butter, sweet almond oil (or apricot kernel oil if you are allergic to almonds and vitamin E).

These body lotions are also perfect to use as a hand cream. Enjoy.

 DERMA RAY TECHNOLOGY

Years ago I was introduced to an amazing device called Derma Ray Technology, patented by Dr. Charles McWilliams.

I had a big cyst in my left breast and the Derma Ray, combined with essential oils, was able to shrink it down by 80% in just 5 sessions. For about 20 minutes, the ray was glided on my armpit and my left chest/breast area. I was so impressed, I thought, "I need to get this electro-frequency proton shower machine in my studio!"

I contacted Dr. McWilliams and was told I could purchase a machine after I received accreditation. One of the ways to achieve this was to become a certified aromatherapist. I found I could learn aromatherapy and the Derma Ray technique by studying at the De Vita Wellness Institute of Living and Learning in Toronto.

In 2005, I was fortunate to get my Derma Ray training with Dr. Sabina M. De Vita, author of the book *Electromagnetic Pollution*, A Hidden Stress to your System. This book details the importance of using natural remedies, including essential oils, to protect yourself from electromagnetic pollution.

For my holistic aromatherapy practitioner intensive diploma program from Langara College, my teacher was Pat Antoniak, a fabulous registered aromatherapist on the West Coast and also a very knowledgeable nurse. Pat encouraged me to become a member of the BCAPA (British Columbia Association of Practicing Aromatherapists), BCAOA (British Columbia Alliance of Aromatherapists) and CFA (Canadian Federation of Aromatherapists). Pat calls her students "aromatherapy angels."

By 2006, I was told I was still the only person on the West Coast of Canada to have the Derma Ray machine.

CELLULAR MASSAGE

The Derma Ray unit is a high-frequency electrotherapy device. In the therapeutic context, high frequencies are frequencies from several hundred kilohertz (kHz) to several thousand megahertz (MHz) per second. Combinations of these frequencies are known as multiplexed high frequencies. The unit sends small multiplexed high frequency electrical signals to the skin via a small glass bulb. The signals are of such a low current that they are scarcely felt, and muscle contractions are not produced.

The waves easily penetrate superficial tissues however, where they have a warming effect, reaching sluggish cells, helping them to absorb oxygen and burn off toxins and cellulite. The photon shower from the glass bulb opens lymphatic blockages and initiates drainage. The sweep frequencies create temporary electrostatic charges, which disperse subdermal stagnant protein that contributes to tissue swelling.

Dr. Eberhart, a high frequency electrotherapy pioneer, referred to the technique as cellular massage.

When you are receiving a Derma Ray session, a vast quantity of photons and electrons are driven into the skin to stimulate enzyme activity, healing responses and tissue oxygenation. During the session you will feel a soothing effect. This tingling effect also feels warm and often increases your vitality and energy level. The unit is adjustable from level one to eleven, customized to the right comfort zone for anyone. I like level five. I find many men settle at level eight, but most women are comfortable at level five or six.

This technology produces ozone at contact and the cleansing effect makes you feel fresh and energized. I usually use a specific blend for targeting your zone of interest. The Derma Ray helps you to absorb the blend of essential oils and increase their healing power in your metabolism. I use this technology on cellulite to help your body flush toxins, reduce swelling and move the lymph. Amazing technology!

In my practice with the device, I find clients enjoy the feeling of stimulated circulation. They report feeling something moving in the physical arena, and a sense that things are shifting. I focus longer on places where I find puffiness. My clients tell me they feel crispy clean afterward—really fresh. It opens the body to receive the essential oils and ushers them into the bloodstream quickly, which is excellent for disinfecting the skin.

For those with oily skin or for heavy smokers, the skin filters out a lot of toxins immediately. Both the client and I can see the thick and gooey toxic residue releasing out of the pores right in front of us. I always follow up with a compress of water to drain the smoke or toxins out of the pores. They don't have to tell me they are a smoker, I know it—I can smell it! This is a good way to clean up the system and detoxify the skin, and it is a very gentle technology.

For clients who have had cancer, I can feel the toxins leaving and smell the medications in their blood as they filter out. At the same time, I have the client focus on whatever they want to release in their lives emotionally. I always make sure to ask for their intention for the session before the massage. I ask if there is any concern or emotional issue they want to release that day. When I use the Derma Ray Technology, I feel they are the Little Soldiers of Light cleaning up for my clients.

Derma Ray helps your oxygen level rise. Oxygenation is excellent for relieving scar tissue and stitches from surgery.

These wounds heal much more quickly with Derma Ray. In addition, it helps with inflammation and all sorts of injuries. If I'm working on an injury, say a muscle, I apply essential oils with a carrier oil, then I use the Derma Ray for 15 to 20 minutes, followed by a warm compress. I can actually feel the lump decreasing inside. Derma Ray is great for sports injuries, such a pitcher who can't lift his arm or athletes who have limitation of motion.

One of my clients, Marci Harriott, is a producer here in Vancouver. She not only loved my aromatherapy massages, but appreciated the reflexology, hot rock massage and the Derma Ray application that came standard with each session. She always told me she felt fully rejuvenated by the time she left my studio.

When Marci first came to me, she was troubled by a snowboarding injury, which, after months of intensive physiotherapy, was simply not getting better. She knew her recovery had hit a plateau and the excessive scar tissue resulted in quite a weak shoulder. Marci came to see me three years after the injury, and when I started to use the Derma Ray Technology on her shoulder, the results were exceptional. Marci reported hearing some crackling during the first session and felt a release in her shoulder, which paved the way to a fuller recovery. After six 90-minute sessions, she revealed that she had regained full strength in her shoulder.

Derma Ray also works on cellulite, helping fat cells shrink and become softer. Clients serious about decreasing cellulite (especially before summertime) come in six weeks in a row in the spring. We focus intently on their cellulite, combining it with an exercise program, cleanse, and a new sport in their lives. I recommend they increase their water intake as well. After six weeks, they notice a big difference. Some of the women get a spray tan on those sexy legs and the next thing I know they've got a boyfriend!

Precautions: Derma Ray cannot be used on anyone who is pregnant or has a pacemaker.

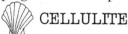 CELLULITE

The first time I massage you, I make sure to assess your "situation" regarding cellulite. When you are on your belly after I've massaged your back, I gently pinch your thighs to evaluate your cellulite level. If a gentle pinch hurts you, it means that your fat cells are getting too hard and compressed and you need to attack the issue. More water, more exercise, and a good cleansing program is mandatory. ⚓ www.cleansing.marinadufort.com

I am always eager to show you how to massage your target zone with the ⚓ Renaissance Glove and the ⚓ Buddha Flush blend. I have seen cellulite on men as well. Remember that cellulite is one of the hardest types of fats to dissolve in the body. It is an accumulation of old fat cell clusters that solidify and harden as the surrounding tissue loses its elasticity. The excess fat is undesirable for two reasons:

1. The added weight puts an extra load on all body systems, including the heart and cardiovascular system and joints (knees, hips and spine).

2. Toxins and petrochemicals like pesticides, herbicides, and metals accumulate in your fatty tissue. This can contribute to hormonal imbalance, neurological problems and a higher risk of cancer. For most of my cancer survivors, I noticed much more impacted cellulite on their thighs before they got sick. So brushing the cellulite regularly is a very good way to help to dissolve it.

Buddha Flush CELLULITE PRODUCTS

Start your day with Buddha Yoga Fresh Lemongrass body gel soap so you can salute the sun while lessening your cellulite. Your circulation is also stimulated very quickly if you massage your thighs with the ✦ **Renaissance Glove** and the super oil blend for cellulite, ✿ *Buddha Flush*. After you dry off from your shower with ✵ *Buddha Yoga Fresh*, apply ✿ *Buddha Flush*. Always make small circular motions towards the heart when you brush. The blend makes you feel warmer on the targeted zone because of the Black Pepper (*Piper nigrum*).

This oil is fantastic for improving your lymphatic flow and activates your circulation. The Grapefruit (*Citrus x paradisi*) is excellent to help water retention and the cellulite runs scared when it senses Grapefruit because it is a very powerful fat burner. Cypress (*Cupressus sempervirens*) is quite beneficial as a powerful lymph decongestant, a fitness booster and one of the best oils if you have varicose veins and spider veins. The jojoba carrier oil keeps the formula fresh and makes your skin silky.

When I lived in Banff, in the Rockies of Alberta, I mountain biked every day, drank tons of green tea and massaged my thighs with essential oils—and I had <u>no cellulite</u>. When I lived in Japan studying acupressure at the Shiatsu Academy of Osaka, I used my charinko (a grandmother-crazy-heavy-black-non-sexy-iron-bike used by everybody for errands) and this dragon of iron was so heavy, oh my gosh. I even gave rides to my friends! I had zero cellulite because of this bike and the Japanese diet, washed down with lots of green tea, and, of course, I used my essential oil *Buddha Flush Blend*. Biking is the enemy of cellulite!

MOTHER NATURE IS THERE FOR YOU

To activate your blood circulation and your lymphatic system, please start to change your lifestyle by escaping outside at least once a day for your precious communion with Mother Nature. I just love my brisk walks in the forest, or on the sea wall of beautiful Vancouver. In the mountains, many hikes are available on the West Coast of British Columbia. Where do you like to walk?

My very popular small motivational inhalers help me breathe more deeply and get an extra "aoumfff" (my favorite onomatope, when a word sounds like what it is). I can't stress enough how vital it is to get out of the house and commune with nature.

Power walking with ❀ **Nose Job Sports** inhaler with Peppermint and Spearmint give me the energy to get it done! Inhale and go walk or go to the gym and get <u>buffed</u>.

Power walking for a short amount of time daily helps my circulation so much. If I have been too busy working, standing on my feet massaging for hours, my circulation gets sluggish. I usually feel my glutes and my abdomen area tingling a lot when I start power walking again. It is a sign that I was getting way too sedentary. It moves my blood, my lymph, and the puffiness in my legs or ankles dissipates very quickly when I exercise by walking or pedaling on the cross-training machine at the gym. I feel the life coming back in my body and it feels so amazing. Yoga is also so good for your lymph. I always make sure that I add some yoga classes into my program. I really enjoy <u>Yin Yoga</u>, an excellent type of yoga to help you to stretch your fascia gently. It helps me connect with my higher spirit. Namaste.

I like to treat myself with a bit of fashion when I exercise. **Spiritual Gangster** (USA) is a clothing line of extremely comfortable funky outfits to wear when you are in your yoga mode. My favorite piece these days is my white tank top that says, "Salute the Sun." I just love wearing it and feeling energized by the words—words are so powerful.

At the end of the day I ask you to elevate your legs higher than your heart for at least ten minutes. You can do that by sitting against the wall in your room with your legs up or by lying down on the bed with a mountain of pillows under your knees and feet. Strike the pose for 10 minutes and feel the puffiness leaving your body. If you are dehydrated, have been standing too long, have menstrual bloating tension or do not exercise on a regular basis, your circulation is stagnant and needs a jumpstart. If you massage ❀ *Buddha Flush* Blend on your ankles they will shrink in size. No more "watermelon feet," only melons in your bra! It is more sexy, hey?

HIGH BLOOD PRESSURE

When your blood pressure is too high, there is a good chance that you are experiencing too much stress, the weight of responsibilities, and possibly too much alcohol, smoking or coffee, a sedentary lifestyle, poor nutrition or obesity. These are all lifestyle ailments. I have many friends who have high blood pressure and one of the best oils to help them to calm down is the beautiful Lavender oil (*Lavendula angustifolia*). They connect very well with this oil, by inhalation or application of the ❀ *Marie-Jeanne de France* lotion, both good ways to take care of the problem.

Lavender is a great hypotensive essential oil. I love using Lavender, Neroli, Bergamot, Chamomile, Ylang Ylang and

Orange to help prevent high blood pressure. The best way to incorporate these oils in your daily life at home or at work is to use a diffuser.

LOW BLOOD PRESSURE

When your blood pressure drops, it means that you are getting exhausted (physically or emotionally). You do not need Lavender essential oil in your life. You need Thyme, Rosemary, Lemon, Ginger, Pine and Clove. Inhale a few drops of these oils mixed with water in a diffuser to help you to feel more energized. Or you can use one oil at a time.

An easy and pleasant way to get the benefit of essential oils is to use an ultrasonic diffuser at home or at work.

DIFFUSING THE OILS

I really like ✴ **THE MIST de Light Ultrasonic Diffuser and Mist Lamp**. This diffuser is different because standard diffusers work by heating essential oils, which can alter or break down the oils. This gadget accomplishes the same task without any changes in the oils through the process of ultrasonic diffusion. It also acts as a humidifier to help freshen the air and keep your skin and nose from getting too dry in the winter. Moist air lessens the transmission of viruses as well.

It comes with soft-colored LED bulbs and ionizes the air that you breathe, creating negative ions, which create positive vibes to elevate your mood. According to Denise Mann, writing for Web MD, ions are molecules that have gained or lost an electrical charge. In nature, air molecules become separated by sunlight, radiation, wind or moving water. You're affected by negative ions on mountaintops and at the beach. They increase serotonin and oxygen flow to the brain. Serotonin is a body chemical that "ups" your mood, relieving depression and stress, and boosting energy. This is the most perfect tool I've found for diffusing your precious essential oils. Remember, negative ions = positive vibes.

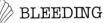 BLEEDING

Just a little word about bleeding. If you cut yourself, the fastest way to stop the bleeding is by using one or two drops on the cut of one of these hemostatic essential oils: Lemon, Geranium, Lime, Eucalyptus, Cypress or Rose. They are amazing they work so fast. I keep some of these oils in my fridge so that if I cut my fingers, I have something to apply on them right away. It is also excellent for stopping nose bleeds. Just put few drops on a tissue and inhale one of these oils to stop the bleeding quickly.

BRUISES

If you bruise easily, the most common reason is a deficiency in vitamin C. The best way to minimize the bruise is to ice it or use a cold compress on the area right away. Then you can apply a few drops of Rosemary or Black Pepper or Ginger mixed with a dash of vegetable oil.

Note: From here on, I refer to the use of vegetable oil several times. This means any edible household oil will do. Rather than using corn or canola oils, however, your best bet is virgin or extra virgin olive oil or grape seed oil.

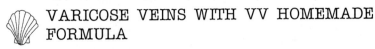 VARICOSE VEINS WITH VV HOMEMADE FORMULA

People who stand all day are more prone to develop varicose veins because their blood cannot circulate. Again, a walk at lunchtime is so vital for you to help the circulation to flow. If you have varicose veins, you probably own support stockings—

they help but do not fix the problem. If you are flying, please make sure you carry a bottle of Peppermint, Cypress, Lemon or Geranium in your purse.

Before you get called to board, go to the washroom to massage a few drops on your ankles and legs in an upward movement towards the heart, then put your contusion special socks on. Wash your hands and go to your flight knowing that this little ritual will save you from getting swollen ankles and legs. Do not touch your eyes with Peppermint on them! At home you can use five drops each of these oils and mix them with two tablespoons of vegetable oil and massage your ankles and legs at night.

VV Homemade Formula: Mix five drops of Peppermint, Cypress, Lemon and Geranium in two tablespoons of vegetable oil. Massage your legs and ankles gently toward the heart.

I also really enjoy mixing three drops of Fennel with three drops of Cypress with three drops of Helichrysum (also called Immortelle) as it is the ultra-respected anti-inflammatory oil. Mix these essential oils together in one tablespoon of vegetable oil then apply on the varicose vein.

 ## COLD/HOT FOOT BATH

Take a footbath with your feet in an ice-cold water bowl with two drops of Lavender for five minutes. Cold water constricts your blood vessels. Then put your feet in another bowl of warm water with two drops of Geranium—the hot water dilates, helping to send the blood back through the body. Then massage very gently the VV formula on your legs and ankles and keep your legs up for ten minutes. <u>Never put pressure on varicose veins.</u>

The skin being your biggest organ, it will reflect on the outside what is going on with you internally. You are in charge of your lifestyle. Your skin is affected by your water intake, your nutrition, stimulants like coffee, tea, alcohol and smoking. It is your responsibility to be mindful of sun exposure, proper sleep, weight gain or weight loss, stress levels, hormonal fluctuations and the amount of medication you are on. So many factors create beautiful balanced skin or dry, oily inflamed skin.

It takes 28 days for your skin layers to come from the dermis to the outer layers of the epidermis. Exfoliating helps to get rid of the dead cells, a very healthy process. When I lived in Japan, I used to go to the Huge Japanese Onsen/Spa called New Japan, where women would soak in different water pools with mineral waters, salt, cold and hot. I would always get the scrubbing session. They give you a plastic J-string to wear while you lie down on the table and get exfoliated by two Japanese girls using soap and salt balls all over your body. Then they hose you down with very cold water. My skin was so happy. I felt so much better after that session. *Domo Arigato!*

In general, the fewer chemicals you use on your face, the better off you are. There are so many brands of skin care in the world. But in my world of aromatherapy for skin care, I am not interested in creating another skin cream. My main focus is to help you to keep your face smiling. I created three facial spritzers to help brighten and raise the vibration of your facial skin.

 ### *Salute the Sun* MORNING ABLUTION

10 ml blend/10 ml spritzer

This beautiful spritzer is like a fresh breeze of very exquisite essential oils to help your skin start the day. The fusion of fresh Lemon (*Citrus limonum*) helps make you stronger. Lemon being the masculine version of orange, it's a very yang essential oil to kick your day into gear with an immunity boost—a beautiful astringent as well.

Then add Neroli (*Citrus aurantium var.amara*), also a more masculine essential oil, it will support you like an angel by lifting your mood for the day. Also, it is such a good oil for any type of skin. Finally, add the very hot Jasmine (*Jasminum officinalis*) because of its aphrodisiac properties and also because it makes your skin softer and supports dry and very sensitive skin.

You can buy the ❀ **Salute the Sun** blend in a 10 ml of Jojoba oil and simply use eight drops of the blend in a 10 ml of water spritzer. Spray every morning and carry with you during the day. Just refill the spritzer with your master blend.

Green Wing AFTERNOON ABLUTION

10 ml blend/10 ml spritzer

This is my ultimate pick-me-up aroma trip to push my face to smile through the afternoon. It is a very invigorating spritzer if you are feeling lethargic at work. Your skin will love it. First of all, the Cypress (*Cupressus sempervirens*) is astringent and will help release your worry. Even your puffy eyes will get better. The Cypress aroma transports me to the forest.

Another ingredient is Lime (*Citrus latifolia*), a wonderful digestive tonic to help with the apathy and lethargy that often happens after lunch. It's a wonderful oil to let go of fatigue and protect you from the flu at work, plus a beautiful oil for controlling excessively oily skin. The Peppermint (*Mentha piperita*) is a super digestive helper and mental clarity and focus guardian that will make your skin feel fresh and free from bacteria.

Get the 10 ml blend with the Jojoba carrier oil and use eight drops per 10 ml spritzer filled with water. Spritz your 🌸 *Green Wing* on your face and feel the love and protection from this aromatherapy angel.

 ## *White Wing* EVENING ABLUTION

10 ml blend/10 ml spritzer

This blend helps restore a natural balance after your evening shower. 🌸 *White Wing* is the best way to make sure that you are clear and open ready for a great night's sleep. Lavender (*Lavandula angustifolia*) supports you to finally relax and let go. It will calm and heal your skin. An antiseptic, it is also called "the mother of the essential oils," because it is recommended for a multitude of ailments. Lavender helps your skin to clean up and cool down before sleep.

The orange (*Citrus sinensis* or *aurantium*) regenerates oily, mature or stressed skin. A very happy essential oil! This blend is powerful, and with the foundation of Sandalwood (*Santalum album*) it is fabulous if your skin is dry or inflamed. You will get the right attention with this oil. Orange radiates a calming vibration to your central nervous system while it helps your skin retain elasticity.

Enjoy the blessing of 🌸 *White Wing* blends at the end of your hectic day or even before you go to bed. Just like Archangel Michael—a great protector during your sleep. Night night!

The world we have created is a product of our thinking; it cannot be changed without changing our thinking.
-Albert Einstein

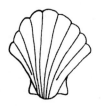

Seashell #5
Annihilate Headaches and
Migraines the Natural Way

How many of you suffer from headaches? And how many of you just automatically reach for the bottle of drugs to deal with it? Raise your hand if you would rather use natural remedies instead!

Did you know that 38% of the population has headaches every two weeks? Headaches are a very common ailment for 85% of the population. You can suffer from general headaches, gastric and hunger headaches, nervous or tension headaches, sinus headaches and hormonal imbalance headaches. Lack of hydration and muscular tension can also cause headaches. Then there are the super migraines, one of the most challenging types of head pain. When you are experiencing headaches, your body is clearly trying to tell you to stop or slow down. Make sure you drink plenty of water. Closing your eyes and taking deep breaths is good for you. I call this the reboot moment for relaxing your neurons!

 GENERAL HEADACHE

I have been carrying Peppermint and Lavender essential oils

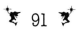

in my purse for a long, long time. When you have a general headache you can inhale the oils straight from the bottle for few minutes for immediate relief of a general headache. If it is a more intense headache, you can put one drop of Lavender and one drop of Peppermint in your left hand, then rub your hands together clockwise to elevate the frequency of your oils. Then place your hands over your nose and breathe… ahhhhhh. Do not touch your eyes!

You can also rub three drops of Lavender and one drop of Peppermint together with one drop of vegetable oil and massage this mini blend around your temples, the base of your skull along the hairline. You can also apply the oils on a tissue and wave it in front of your nose. Please pinch between the thumb and index in the web of your hand to stimulate the release of toxins. This is a super popular meridian headache release point in Shiatsu massage, even more powerful for fast relief if combined with Peppermint and Lavender.

 GASTRIC HEADACHE REMEDIES

Let's say for example that you are invited to a Chinese restaurant for a birthday dinner. You eat and then suddenly you have a headache caused possibly by MSG (MSG is a flavor enhancer) that you usually do not consume. Or you just have an instant headache if you eat the food that is wrong for your metabolism. Mix one drop of Lavender, two drops of Peppermint and one drop of Rosemary. Now this synergy blend is ready to be used. Use one drop of that blend on a tissue and inhale gently. You can also use three drops of the blend in a steam inhalation. Boil water, pour it in a cup and add three drops of the blend. Inhale the steam slowly. This is a great way to feel better <u>fast</u>.

TENSION OR NERVOUS HEADACHE RECIPE

Combine one drop of Chamomile and three drops of Lavender with one drop of vegetable oil, then massage one drop of the blend over your temples, the base of your skull and along the hairline. If you feel more adventurous, you can create a belly blend with three drops of Lavender, two drops of Lemon and one drop of Geranium in one teaspoon of vegetable oil and then massage your abdomen in a clockwise direction. This relaxes your solar plexus and the tension in your head goes away smoothly.

 ## SINUS HEADACHE SOOTHER

If you are getting congested and sick, this combination of oils in a steam inhalation method works like a charm. Mix one drop of Peppermint and one drop of Thyme with three drops of Rosemary in a cup of boiled water, then inhale lightly for few minutes. Now you can breathe again. Make sure you inhale slowly and that the water is not super hot. Always be cautious and aware of the perfect temperature for your nose, and be sure to close your eyes when you inhale.

If you are in a hurry, just mix one drop of Eucalyptus, one drop of Geranium and two drops of Rosemary together, then pour one drop of that blend on a tissue and inhale again and again and again.

If you are sick at home, you can go for the full-on super home made *Nurse Blend* consisting of two drops of Eucalyptus, five drops of Geranium, three drops of Peppermint and five drops of Rosemary. Then shake well and mix five drops of *Nurse Blend* with one teaspoon of vegetable oil, and massage your neck, behind and in front of the ears, under the nose, on the forehead and over the cheekbones so your sinuses get the help to filter out bacteria.

 ## MIGRAINE RELIEF

When you are getting a migraine, you need to chill and stop. Does your head feel like it's going to explode? Promise yourself you will be gentle with yourself today. Your body is asking for gentleness and caring. Mix five drops of Eucalyptus, five drops of Grapefruit and five drops of Lavender in your left hand then massage your hands together, cup your nose and inhale. Inhale and inhale and have a quiet time—perhaps go relax in your car at lunchtime if you are working to soothe that migraine.

 ## HEADACHE GOOONE

Headache Gooone super blend is a simple way to get rid of a headache naturally. *Headache Gooone* can be used for massaging your neck, skull, jaw line, hairline, abdomen and ankles. Massage is fantastic if you have a hormonal headache, and one drop under your nose is great as well. This already-made "just for you" blend has a jojoba carrier oil and is placed in a 10 ml bottle to help you big-time. The super cooling and analgesic spritzer form is very effective. Just spritz it, walk in it and inhale with joy.

LAVENDER

Lavender: middle note, calming. Botanical name: *Lavandula angustifolia, Lavandula officinalis.*

Safety data: It is better to use in the last four months of your pregnancy. It also helps to lower your blood pressure, so if you already have low blood pressure you should not use it. Less is more. Non-toxic, non-irritant, non-sensitizing.

For me, lavender is a very powerful therapeutic essential oil. It is fantastic to calm and rebalance your nervous system. In Medieval times, people were divided in two clans of Lavender promoters: those who associated it with love and chastity, and those who believed in its aphrodisiac property.

Lavender has been used as a folk remedy for so long and for so many things. The whole plant is highly aromatic: every time I see Lavender, I gently crush the linear leaves or the violet blue flowers in my hands and sniff sniff sniff like I am the happiest dog on this planet! If I were not so shy I would roll over in it!

I have been to Lavender fields in France and had the chance to pluck Lavender flowers in La Marmande near Bordeaux at ✴ "Le petit Bardeche," thanks to the hospitality of my Norwegian friends, the Rorvik and Vigander families. Check out their website at http://www.holidaycottagesandvillas.com.

Merci Mon Dieu pour la Lavande de France! Wonderful for headache relief. Mother of all oils.

PEPPERMINT

Peppermint: Top note. Botanical name: *Mentha piperita*.

Safety data: Not compatible if you are on homeopathic treatment. Not to be used if you are pregnant or breastfeeding, as it will stop your milk production. Possibility of sensitization because of high level of menthol. Less is more. Not to be used on babies and infants.

Peppermint is a great analgesic and it has been used for centuries for mental focus and concentration, freshening breath, digestive purposes and headaches. It is a wonderful anti-inflammatory. In her book ✳ *Aromatherapy*, Roberta Wilson researches the origin of the Peppermint name, writing "In Roman mythology, when Pluto professed his love to the nymph Mentha, his wife Persephone was so jealous that she crushed Mentha into dust on the ground. Pluto, unable to change her back, transformed her into a Peppermint plant and gave her a fresh fragrance so that she would smell sweet whenever stepped on."

When I worked in the film industry, people would know I was around because I always used Peppermint on myself, to be in the zone. It wakes you up full on! I love using this oil by inhalation or by topical application to reduce throbbing pain.

SPEARMINT

Spearmint: Top note. Botanical name: *Mentha spicata*.

Safety data: should be avoided during pregnancy, and avoid using on babies and infants. Same as Peppermint, it disrupts breast milk production and will interfere with homeopathic remedies.

For me, Spearmint is the little cousin of Peppermint, possessing mainly the same properties with less power. I love using Spearmint in a spritzer form to alleviate headaches and migraines. It is the Juicy Fruit® chewing gum smell for cooling down your brain. Very uplifting, it blends well with Peppermint and Lavender.

I want to share with you the great story of Christian White, the ultimate sceptic for natural remedies now the happy consumer of aromatherapy.

"To say my life is hectic would be an understatement. My passion is helping people and I have been a financial consultant for 10+ years. I look at every angle to try and make an efficient use of my business and my time... and in that quest I came across Marina!

Throughout my life I have been a sceptic of anything that can't be scientifically proven, so when I first met Marina and was introduced to aromatherapy I was still a cynic. My initial session with Marina involved relaxation massage/aromatherapy, all due to the fact I was working a lot running my business, suffering from headaches and a minor back injury. I had tried chiropractic treatment, different massage therapies and also acupuncture. None of these approaches worked for me.

Through Marina I finally discovered the natural help of Peppermint and Spearmint essential oils using her Inhaler called **Nose Job Sports**. Here is my story...Spending many hours researching and seeing clients, I found myself reaching for things to boost my energy in the early to late afternoon (especially on long days). I would usually reach for a Starbucks coffee to get me the extra mile. I found that this was a great way for a short period of time and then I would crash. Marina suggested that I try her **Nose Job** Spearmint inhaler. I had my doubts. However, now I no longer reach for the caffeinated drinks—I use Marina's inhaler. I keep one in my office, one at home, and one in my car. Whenever I need to perk up or get ready for a serious meeting, I use the inhaler to clear my nasal passages and it really helps me focus!

A funny thing happened to me a few months back while studying at the Vancouver Public Library. I was close to wrapping up my studying for the day and found myself reaching for **Nose Job** inhaler as I was getting fairly tired. At this point I was sniffing the inhaler every 15 minutes or so...I also noticed that the security guard had walked passed me quite a few times... and each time I also looked at him to see what he was doing.

On his seventh or eighth pass I picked up my inhaler and took a quick whiff! He abruptly stopped, pointed his finger at me and accused me of using drugs! I laughed... he did not. I told him what it was and showed him the label. It was only then that he got a good giggle.

I am now an avid aromatherapy user because Marina makes sure I release tension (I go to the gym at five AM five days a week and I play golf). She makes sure I see her every 21 days for my two hours of relaxation, with an aromatherapy session and foot bath detox. I am also losing weight and getting stronger with my higher energy levels.

If you are a sceptic, cynic or have any doubts about the healing powers of aromatherapy used along with professional massage treatments/detox, I would strongly advise you to try Marina's secret recipe. I did and have not looked back since.

Christian White, Division Director, Christian.White@investorsgroup. com

Enjoy your ❀ **Headache Gooone** blend or spritzer. To avoid headaches, make sure you drink plenty of water every day and take the time to breath deeply and bring oxygen into your body. Vow to be a shallow breather no more!

 *The Universe will knock itself out to supply your wishes.*
-Abraham-Hicks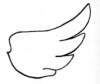

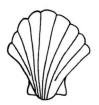

Seashell #6
Quick, Easy and Powerful Solutions to Constipation and Bloating, Acid Reflux and Parasites

The digestive system, what a beautiful system it is—when it is working well. The GI tract (gastrointestinal tract) starts at the mouth and ends up in the rectum, measuring about 25 feet long. Hopefully for you, the journey your food takes to travel along that route is a smooth one.

CONSTIPATION

As a child I was very sensitive and usually constipated. I would sit for hours on the toilet seat waiting for the miracle to happen. Why? Nutrition for sure was my big problem. I never liked vegetables and fruit back then. I grew up in Quebec and I was addicted to gravies, fried food, meats, sugar, dairy and breads. Water was not the most popular choice for me either. It is only by studying nutrition over the years that I am now cleared, finally, of my problem.

Massive amounts of liquid travel my GI tract every day. I love starting my day with a glass of fresh water mixed with lemon juice to make sure I get my pipes all cleaned up with alkaline-forming lemon. I also enjoy massaging my belly in a clockwise direction with vegetable oil (one tablespoon) and Patchouli (*Pogostemon cablin*) (five drops). This is an excellent intestinal cleansing oil. The bonus? It is also an aphrodisiac...

🐚 CONSTIPATION BELLY RUB

Drinking a cup of hot water will help prepare the belly to let go. When you are at home or traveling and you have an issue with constipation, you can mix three drops of Sandalwood (*Santalum album*), three drops of Black Pepper (*Piper nigrum*), three drops of Ginger (*Zingiber officinalis*) and three drops of Grapefruit (*Citrus x paradisi*) in two tablespoons of vegetable oil.

Rub this blend in a circular motion on your belly and just feel the peristalsis waking up. The wave-like motion of the muscle contractions in your GI tract will begin. Halleluiah! The material is getting propelled.

When a client is on the massage table I ask them how their digestion is these days, and depending on what they say I offer them my "Abdomen Soak Blend" to alleviate their discomfort. "Abdomen Soak Flow" helps the GI tract become more active.

🐚 CONSTIPATION: ❀ *Flow* ABDOMEN SOAK

This blend contains Sandalwood (*Santalum album*). It is such a relaxing and comforting oil. As a child, my dear stepmother Huguette, who now studies shamanistic philosophy, told me that I could have been holding onto my past too much when I was not "regular." It makes sense to me now, and Sandalwood helps to let go of the past that can sometimes be a burden.

The other oil in this blend is three drops of Black Pepper (*Piper nigrum*). The super antidote to help you to open the road like a faithful snowplow, this oil is very powerful for moving the circulation in general. Then you add three drops of Ginger (*Zingiber officinalis*). Ginger was my favorite thing to eat in huge quantities when I lived in Japan. I ate a lot of sushi and I really knew the importance of masking the fish smell, but there is great therapeutic value to adding ginger to your digestive system. Ginger oil is super-concentrated and really calms down any problems in the belly. For people with constipation issues, it is truly divine.

Now for the citrus touch, three drops of Grapefruit (*Citrus x paradisi*). I just <u>love</u> the citrus family. Grapefruit is fresh and good for uplifting your mood and dissolving resistance in your body. I mix these oils in a 10 ml bottle of quality Apricot Kernel carrier oil because this oil has anti-inflammatory properties.

I like to use eight drops of this blend on my clients' bellies, massaging it clockwise with warm stones, then applying a hot compress for ten minutes. We usually laugh at all the noises and sounds your colon starts to make. Do not be surprised if you have to go to the washroom right after your session!

Fennel, Marjoram, Juniper, Cardamom, Peppermint, Spearmint, Rosemary and all the citrus oils are also excellent to get some action in your elimination department. When you need it, you can always mix any one of each of these single oils with one tablespoon of vegetable oil and massage it on your belly.

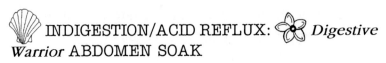 INDIGESTION/ACID REFLUX: *Digestive Warrior* ABDOMEN SOAK

You usually feel the burning pain in your chest signifying a mean heartburn, after a meal, once the stomach acid moves up past the sphincter under your sternum. This is called acid reflux, and usually occurs when the muscle tone in the sphincter is lost, causing it to remain open. The best way to treat it ASAP is to rub your upper abdominal area with:

Eucalyptus (*Eucalyptus globulus*)	2 drops
Peppermint (*Mentha piperita*)	1 drop
Sweet Fennel (*Foeniculum vulgare var. dulce*)	2 drops

Mixed with a teaspoon of Jojoba oil.

Again, if you do not want to carry these essential oils in your luggage just make sure you bring the already blended *Digestive Warrior* Abdomen Soak (Eucalyptus, Peppermint and Sweet Fennel with Jojoba). When you suffer from heartburn, you just have to massage eight drops of the blend on your upper abdominal area (right below your belly button) and apply a warm compress on it for ten minutes.

IRRITABLE BOWEL SYNDROME (IBS)

I have friends who suffer from IBS. When they have too much stress in their lives, they have a war zone in the small and large bowels, with very painful spasms and pain in the lower abdomen, accompanied by diarrhea. For that condition, I really like the use of Petitgrain (*Citrus aurantium var. amara*) (three drops). From the citrus family, it is an extremely safe oil. It is effective for pain and spasms—a fast sedative and calming emergency oil. You can mix it with Peppermint (*Mentha piperita*) (three drops), the classic digestive helper, and Geranium (*Pelargonium graveolens*) (three drops) with one tablespoon of vegetable oil. Apply on your belly and place a nice warm compress there for five minutes. The pain and spasms should subside and your intestine will calm down nicely.

GASTRIC FLATULENCE

Okay! Now I can talk about farts with joy. Because I changed the diapers of my two lovely brothers, I can assure you that this little section is very important. Why does farting seem so funny, especially more for guys than girls? First of all, a lot of my clients did not want to give me permission to release any info regarding their trumpet zone. They said it was too stinky to talk about. Well, if you are afflicted with this problem, your loved ones already know about it and surely you all suffer from it. Deal with it ASAP. If you are a stinky chronic farter, please try my magic recipe for this serious matter. By the way girls do not fart... they release tension! Ha, ha, ha!

GAS: *Belly Zen* ABDOMEN SOAK

Add five drops of Coriander (*Coriandrum sativum*) it is excellent to deal with the situation, then five drops of Fennel (*Foeniculum vulgare var. dulce*)—it is your second defense of choice, and five drops of Frankincense (*Boswellia carteri*), which is super classy. You then mix with two tablespoons of vegetable oil. Rub the solution on your abdomen and gain your respect back!

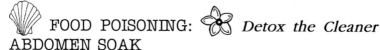 FOOD POISONING: *Detox the Cleaner* ABDOMEN SOAK

If you are a traveler and you enjoy experimenting with local food like a good epicurean, this is a blend to take with you in your suitcase. Because of your adventurous nature, there is a good possibility that you can be affected by something that is "off," not fresh or just does not agree with your system. You do not want to take the chance of this happening.

For food poisoning, make sure you drink plenty of fluid and rest and massage your tummy with:

Lemon (*Citrus limonum*)	5 drops
Lavender (*Lavandula angustifolia*)	5 drops
Geranium (*Pelargonium graveolens*)	5 drops
Ginger (*Zingiber officinalis*)	5 drops
Thyme (*Thymus vulgaris*)	5 drops

Mix these 25 drops in two tablespoons of vegetable oil and apply ***Detox the Cleaner*** Abdomen Soak with a hot compress for ten minutes.

Parasites in Me? No Way! Abdomen Soak

If you eat raw fish, sushi and all, you probably carry little friends called parasites. I suggest a soothing abdomen soak with:

Clove (*Syzygium aromaticum*)	5 drops
Ginger (*Zingiber officinalis*)	5 drops
Eucalyptus (*Eucalyptus globulus*)	5 drops
Peppermint (*Mentha piperita*)	5 drops
Lavender (*Lavandula angustifolia*)	5 drops

Mix these 25 drops in two tablespoons of vegetable oil over the tummy and apply the hot compress Parasite Abdomen Soak for ten minutes.

When you are traveling in a tropical country, you can stave off tummy troubles by applying these abdomen soaks every night as a preventive measure. Lying flat on my back on the washroom floor of an hotel in Indonesia is not how I travel anymore. I've been there, so I really encourage you to be super proactive regarding spoiled food in your system!

When I lived in Japan I fell in love with an Australian surfer from Perth who was living with an Aussie group of hot surfers in Bali. I traveled with him to Indonesia and I loved being immersed in the Indonesian culture. They are very community and family oriented. While they are tight in that way, they pay attention to personal physical boundaries. If a cousin has a problem they all sit down and figure it out. They have rituals and ceremonies for so many things. When you go shopping, they burn incense and pray before they open their stores. It's important for them to have someone with the right energy enter their shop; it sets the tone for the day. They would invite me into their store when I was hurrying to the beach, pleading "We need you!" They are superstitious about not having sales, so the earlier in the day if they get someone to walk in, the more relieved they are. Of course I walked in and I loved the exotic incense smell.

Unfortunately, my dear Aussie friends and I got really sick from a pizza (should have stuck to the classic Indonesian nasi goreng rice meal) while I was there. And that was the day I was flying back to Japan!

It didn't help that dairy products in general are also too harsh for me. I got sick to my stomach almost as soon as I ate the pizza. I was so dizzy, I passed out on the floor of the washroom in the airport where an American good Samaritan woman found me. Somehow I managed to show her my flight information. She told me she would help me and then disappeared. Next thing I knew, she picked me up, put me in a wheelchair and pushed me through the airport as they were saying my name over the PA system. She wheeled me right up the steaming tarmac so I could board my plane to Osaka back to Shiatsu school. Thank you, my angel friend. If I hadn't made that flight, I wouldn't have had money to buy another ticket.

Thank God my seat was in the front row. In Japan, they do not let you on airplanes if you are sick, so I had to hide it as best I could, when all I wanted to do was slump onto the floor and curl up into a ball. Once on the plane, I covered my belly with peppermint essential oils, smelled the bottle of Peppermint constantly and I drank hot water with lemon the whole trip. My greatest wish was not to get sick on anybody for the next six hours. I did not have my essential oil travel kit back then… I wish! But not long after that I started adding oils to my travel apothecary.

Because I want you to be prepared for anything, I have made it easy, combining a home first aid kit for your family and a travel kit for anything from a car camping trip to exploring exotic places around the globe.

I really want to make sure that you understand the power of essential oils in your first aid kit. Always travel with these essential oils—they will empower your health:

MARINA MERMAID FIRST AID and TRAVEL KIT

Clove (*Syzygium aromaticum*)
Eucalyptus (*Eucalyptus globulus*)
German Chamomile (*Matricaria chamomilla*)

Geranium (*Pelargonium graveolens*)

Ginger (*Zingiber Officinalis*)

Grapefruit (*Citrus x paradisi*)

Lavender (*Lavandula angustifolia*)

Lemon (*Citrus limonum*)

Lemongrass (*Cymbopogon citratus*)

Patchouli (*Pogostemon patchouli*)

Peppermint (*Mentha piperita*)

Tea tree (*Melaleuca alternifolia*)

Thyme (*Thymus vulgaris*)

These 13 essential oils are my favorite single oils to carry.

 ## MERMAID TRAVEL SECRET SEASHELL

Usually the first thing I do when I arrive at my hotel after a long flight is put Lemon and Peppermint on a tissue and place it over the air conditioning duct. Then I blast the place for 15 minutes so my room is purified. I also carry a small spritzer bottle so I can mix my favorite oils with water and spray my pillow and the sheets before I go to bed.

 ## PET LOVERS HEALTHY MASSAGE

I love pets. When I babysit them, I always massage them with the blend I call *Doggy Styles*. Because pets carry parasites as well, you, your family and your pets will benefit highly from this preventative and proactive routine. I sit the pets on my lap so they face forward and then I massage them with my formula, comprised of Citronella, Lavender and Tea Tree oil with an Apricot Kernel oil carrier. I do this in a nice gentle motion starting behind their ears and gently rubbing their spine to the tail for a good five minutes. This quality time routine will make small dogs sedated and very happy, and it's great to perform in the evening. It also works in the morning before you leave for work if your pet suffers from separation anxiety. They love it. Promise.

 ## BLOATED?

That is how I feel when I eat in a restaurant and I get carried away by having way too much fun laughing and talking and socializing while I am trying to chew my food—bloated! I am usually a very slow eater and I am always the last to finish my meal. When I dine out, I carry my bottle of Peppermint in my purse without fail. I massage a few drops in my hands and I rub my bloated belly when I've had too much. If I am with friends, I do it right there under the table because it will take care of bloat very quickly. I usually order a Peppermint hot tea to make sure I get the situation under control. I am crazy that way—if it is healthy and good for me I want it <u>now</u>!

A lot of people who know me would say that Peppermint oil usually arrives before I do. My chiropractor told me the other day that it is his favorite scent... almost like an aphrodisiac. Oh my goodness, I can only imagine him running wildly after his wife in a Peppermint field! The point is, people smell me before they see me. How cool is that? I would rather smell of essential oils. They are good for you, without side effects. They keep you high, and safely and naturally healthy!

I feel that I could go on about digestive problems for many pages, but I just want you to start to experiment with these basic recipes for now.

There is a remedy for every illness
to be found in nature.
-Hippocrates

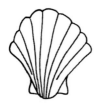

Seashell #7
The Natural Flu Shot to Boost Your Immunity to Colds, Influenza, Asthma and Seasonal Allergies

Basically, when you have a flat tire you stop, put a patch on the hole, and then ride on it until it goes flat again. Eventually you buy a brand new tire. Immunity is like the tire. The patches over the holes are like the man-made drugs that mask the symptoms—they help, but only for a while. Your goal is to have four amazing top-of-the-line new tires that provide you with a feeling of security and strength. It's better to build up your immunity with essential oils because immunity is everything. When you have health, you are rich.

As a baby born in the sixties, I did not get the breast milk, I got the formula. As a child, I had repetitive tonsillitis, allergies and hay fever, and I got really sick of being sick. My body had weak immunity and a compromised respiratory system. I remember playing with Q-tips in front of the mirror trying to get rid of those yellow patches on my tonsils, symbols of my weakness. It was difficult not to gag trying to dislodge the gunk on the back of my throat.

I was a teenager when the doctor suggested surgery. I did not know then that tonsils are the soldiers of my immune system. When you are still living home under the rule of your parents, what the doctor says is the truth. Living in Quebec, doctors are gods over anything else.

So off I went for my first anesthetic surgery at 16 years old. I tried to convince myself that my immunity would get better after the removal of my weak tonsils. If I had known then that the problems of unresolved communication issues were lodged in my throat chakra area (my mother and I did not talk for a year) maybe I could have saved my tonsils by speaking my truth to her.

When she came to see me after the surgery holding a teddy bear in her hands from the hospital gift shop, I thought it was very sweet of her. I appreciated her very much for showing me love that day. She is a strong, controlling Leo and I am a very hot burning Aries—not the best combo when you are in teenage angst full-force and ready to leave the nest. So my weak tonsils were gone and I decided that it was a new beginning for my renewed health. I love you, mom.

But even with my best intentions, after this medical intervention I still had hay fever madness. I went to France for one month with my friends Elise and Sylvie, and it was a challenging experience.

I tried all the antihistamine drugs in the world, but I still had hay fever like crazy, as I tried to visit the beautiful

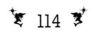 114

castles of Loire, Chenonceau and Chateaux de Versailles. Try enjoying Aix-en-Provence, the kingdom of Lavender fields and honeybees, when you are 17 and you are just so allergic that you just want to jump off the Eiffel Tower to make the discomfort stop! How ironic is that? I saved my money for a year for my first European trip and there I was, trying to enjoy the beautiful French countryside, but not able to see and feel and smell and appreciate it because I was stuffed, irritated, sneezy and puffy! I did not know about essential oils then.

When I was 21, I noticed one thing about myself that probably applies to most people. When I do not align with my message or my own truth, or make it known to people, my immunity gets low and I become sick with allergies and bronchitis. The last time this happened was when I was dating this very hot (but not so good for me) man and I was financially so depleted and so stressed that I was sick for an entire month. Wow! I realize now how much I was lacking the power of expressing my feelings, and how low energy, negative thinking and the constant stream of pessimistic inner dialogue meant sickness for me.

I finally discovered essential oils at 26 years old. I wish I had met a great aromatherapist when I was a child! So now you understand my precious desire to make sure that you start to use essential oils in your daily life with your family. Do this and I know that you will get healthier, my friend.

Your immune system is the most important system in your body when it comes to preventing disease. A weak immune system increases your chances of becoming ill with any type of infection. Low immunity can be detected if these signs are present in your life:

115

Do you suffer from frequents colds and flu?

Do you suffer from chronic infections?

Do you have frequent cold sores?

When your army of immunity soldiers are not well trained and strategically positioned, you have a good chance of being invaded by the bad guys. Let's start here with common sense.

One thing that I have been sharing with all my beautiful clients and friends is to use the alkaline soldier in the morning. For years, I have started my day with a glass of water and lemon juice (one tablespoon), the ultimate alkaline elixir of the gods.

Lemon is acidic, but when absorbed in the stomach it turns alkaline (9.9 ph positive) and really helps your body to clean up its pipes! It assists your liver and gallbladder by flushing out the ducts. When you ingest meat, let's say beef for example, it turns your stomach an acidic negative 34.5 ph. By contrast, cucumber turns alkaline in your stomach to +31.5ph. To make it easy, you can buy bottles of organic pressed lemon juice. At the spa, I like to add a slice of lemon floating in the water. It's beautiful. Also, adding cucumber slices to water is a fantastic way to maintain positive alkalinity levels in your system.

Make sure you consult the list of alkaline and acidic forming food in the Appendix.

When your body is alkaline, there is no room for inflammation. Inflammation has been shown to be a source of conditions such as cancer, Alzheimer's, heart disease, diabetes, arthritis, lupus, multiple sclerosis, and even autism. There is inflammation that you know about because you feel it, such as acute pain in your knees or shoulders, and then there is the silent kind that you don't even notice—chronic inflammation in your vascular system.

Is there a way to curb inflammation in your body? Yes, by avoiding foods you are allergic to (get tested!), as well as environmental toxins (mold, heavy metals in vaccines and dental fillings, air pollution, etc.). Inflammation also occurs as a result of chronic stress and trauma, infections (especially hidden infections, both bacterial and viral), unhealthy diets and lack of exercise. The good news is you can become healthy, disease-resistant and energetic by eating the right foods that reduce inflammation. Avoid processed foods, sugar, carbs, grain-fed meat and farmed fish and increase your intake of omega-3s with wild salmon, walnuts, flax and chia seeds and other omega-3 rich seeds, wild game, free-range meats and leafy greens.

COLDS AND FLU

In the USA, $1 billion a year is spent on non-prescriptions drugs for colds and flu. I am a big advocate of letting the cold and flu run its own natural course, with the help of essential oils, to allow the mucous to expel the toxins, virus and infection out of your system. Statistics report that a typical person will be subjected to cold or flu viruses three times a year. Personally, I do not like being part of any statistic. Because of my professional choice of career, I have been blessed with the best army of soldiers of love, the sacred essential oils.

Every time I give a massage treatment, I receive the benefit through my hands, and my body gets the extra immune boost from the aromatherapy. I use essential oils every day of my life and I am rarely sick now... I would say maybe only once every two years, generally in the springtime. Why? Because my immunity is now so much stronger. Also if you are suffering from fibromyalgia you can benefit from aromatherapy to help you to lower your stress level.

After battling fibromyalgia for 20 years and trying many forms of therapy,
I realized that relaxation with aromatherapy massages with Lavender
and Citrus essential oils was the answer. After a session with Marina,
I feel relaxed, rejuvenated with no flair-ups.
Thank you, Marina.

Kelly Hairdresser
Owner, Bliss the Studio
<u>*www.blissthestudio.com*</u>
North Vancouver, B.C. Canada

SOLUTIONS FOR COLDS AND FLU

More than 150 viruses can cause a cold, an infection of your upper respiratory tract. If you live in a cold climate with snow in the winter, there are more chances for you to get infected. The first symptom is the sore throat—feeling like it is on fire with razor blade itchiness.

As soon as you feel this, it's time to swallow a clove of garlic with water. This is the first natural antibiotic that my body enjoys. I do not bite it, I just wolf it down with water. Because garlic's main compound is allicin, it makes it a fantastic antibacterial/antifungal/immuno stimulant and antioxidant star.

Then for an immune booster, I use the best oil of Wild Oregano (*origanum vulgare*) under the tongue. Make sure it is organic, and that the level of carvacrol (this is the type of phenol, the antiseptic agent) is elevated (86%). Even if it is mixed with organic extra virgin olive oil or coconut extract, it tastes like a whole farm of hay bales but it does the best cleanup for killing germs, fungus and bacteria right away. It is an excellent assistant to fight the bad guys for you naturally.

I like to buy two bottles at the health food store and I know I am safe for the wintertime.

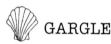

GARGLE

I also gargle with salt and warm water and use a nasal syringe or neti pot with saline water to clean my sinuses in the morning. I love to gargle with water and three drops of tea tree oil as well.

DIFFUSE

I have a diffuser both at home and at work, and I use different blends to purify the air. I love having a pleasant bath with essential oils and solar salts (salt water dried in the sun), also known as sea salts, Himalayan salts, Epsom salts and/or magnesium oil. My favorite choice to diffuse in the air to dispel cold and flu are Eucalyptus, Lavender, Cedarwood, Thyme, Chamomile, Peppermint, Cypress, Lemon, Pine and Myrrh.

LUXURIOUS HEALTHY DETOX BATH

I love having a healthy bath with either solar, Himalayan or Epsom salts with magnesium oil and other essential oils. I mix one cup of salt with one drop of each essential oil of Lavender, Ginger, Frankincense, Lemon, Thyme and Tea Tree with a tablespoon of carrier oil dissolved in my bath. I soak for 20 minutes maximum. Ahhhhhhhh!

THIS SUPER SPEEDY SORE THROAT REMEDY DOUBLES AS A THROAT AND CHEST RUB

I also like to mix one drop of Peppermint, one drop of Lavender, one drop of Eucalyptus, one drop of Tea Tree and one drop of Pine together with one tablespoon of Apricot Kernel oil and massage it on my throat and chest area. Then I put a warm compress on my throat for five minutes and I feel the heat, the essential oils at work. The more infected you are, the hotter it seems to feel. I love it when it gets hot and steaming because I imagine the toxins and bacteria screaming and trying to escape in a panic. BAM, tag you are hit, GOOONE! Then I just rest for one hour and the sore throat is over.

SOLUTIONS AT WORK

I worked on film sets for years and I just had to make an inhaler, not just for me but for my co-workers as well. We all work in such close proximity that if one person gets sick, then the other 150 crew members have a good chance of getting infected. I enjoy a great, simple easy way to inhale through a neat and compact small hygienic inhaler that I call ❀ *Nose Job*. I now have a lot of addicted members in the film biz community. I am a proud pusher of natural remedies!

❀ *Nose Job Crystal Clear* is loaded with Eucalyptus essential oil, which is an excellent decongestant, and ❀ *Nose Job Sports* does a great job of keeping you alert and awake when you are working nightshifts. Peppermint and Spearmint oils are encapsulated in that blend. It's excellent for using at the gym when you are looking for that extra <u>aoumfff</u> of energy needed to pump your dumbbells. All of the cold and detox bath remedies mentioned will also help you.

INFLUENZA

Influenza, which we call the flu or *la grippe*, is also extremely annoying. It makes you feel lethargic, with fever and aches and pains, and it usually lasts longer than the typical cold. Over-the-counter drugs are really good at suppressing the symptoms, but by doing this they block your body's self-defense mechanisms. What you want is "the works," and the essential oils are the best mechanics for the job because they address the source of the problem and build up your immunity.

 ## INHALATION

My favorite choice to ease a cold and get breathing again is a blend of Tea Tree, Eucalyptus and Pine essential oils in a diffuser. I really recommend the chest rubs as well.

 ## CHEST RUB

As a kid I was addicted to Vicks® VapoRub® over-the-counter ointment. Unfortunately, the therapeutic grade essential oil of menthol and blend of Eucalyptus oils in the product is now synthetic (as it's cheaper to make). So I make my own chest rubs. I make it easy for you to massage your chest, throat, back, and feet with my blend called ❀ *Breath Booster* rub: Pine, Eucalyptus Globulus and Tea Tree with Jojoba oil. Go to bed with that sacred doctor and feel the immunity coming back into your life force the next morning.

One of my clients, a high-powered lawyer, started getting massages once a month and found that she didn't get her usual winter cold or flu. Now she would never think of skipping a session because feeling good and healthy is her priority. She uses the ❀ *Nose Job* inhaler at work and has bottles of Lavender, Peppermint, Eucalyptus and Lemon essential oils at home and in her desk at work.

Another client, my dear Romy, is able to boost her immunity with the help of essential oils as well.

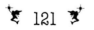

"A year after a double mastectomy, I slowly accepted my body and the psychological scars that the cancer operation had caused.

It was my daughter, who had met Marina, who suggested and paid for lymph drainage massage. The massage and the aromatherapy that Marina gave me improved my energy and gave me a new outlook on life. I since have been back for many more treatments—especially the aromatherapy stone massage.

On another occasion, I had a very bad cold. First, I did not want to take the massage treatment, worrying to infect Marina. However, she suggested I should come, it would not bother her at all. The healing massage with all the special oils and Derma Ray treatment helped me tremendously and my cold soon disappeared.

I can highly recommend Marina and wish her lots of success in her endeavor.

Romy Reimann

B.C. Canada

ALLERGIES

An allergy is a hypersensitive reaction to a normally harmless substance, which we then label as an allergen. Common allergens are feathers, pollen, house dust, animal dander, mites, insecticides, powders and a variety of foods. Some allergies cause respiratory symptoms; others cause headaches, fever, diarrhea, vomiting and stomachaches. Respiratory allergies are chronic or seasonal.

When you have allergies, you are either dealing with a stuffy or runny nose, itchy skin and eyes, sneezing, or red watery eyes. You are also irritable with no patience. Your body recognizes the allergen and your immune system releases chemicals called histamines to fight the invader. It is like going at war with others and against yourself.

 HAY FEVER INHALATION REMEDIES

Hay fever for me is the most annoying allergy ever. Now that I discovered how effective essential oils are through inhalation, it is the best method for me when I have allergies. I use one drop of Peppermint with one drop of Lavender neat in my left hand. I massage my hands and cup them over my nose and inhale this awesome bliss. I also like to put the drops on a tissue that I carry in my pocket during the day. This little trick really saved my life while working on a Western with Tom Berenger called *Peacemakers*, with horses, dogs, hay, dust, gunshots, and a record summer heatwave. When shooting at night, they added a smoke machine for atmosphere and the film crew got an added dose of nose and eye aggravation. By the end of the shoot, the whole crew was on Peppermint and Lavender essential oils, giving thanks to aromatherapy.

 ASTHMA

Asthma is a very common respiratory disease; it affects the trachea and the bronchial tubes, causing them to become inflamed and plugged with mucus. The airways become so narrow that the air going to your lungs is restricted and you have difficulty breathing. Asthma is very common in children and young adults. Typical symptoms of an asthma attack are coughing, wheezing, tight chest and difficulty breathing.

The causes are typically chemicals, drugs, smoke, dust, food additives, pollution, mold, stress, anxiety, and weather changes (too dry or too humid). I recommend staying away from steam inhalation remedies, which include the oils of Eucalyptus,

Rosemary and Peppermint if you have asthma. The steam is so intensified when your head is over a hot pot covered with a towel. These vibrant oils are a bit strong for this method and could trigger an attack.

 ## SOLUTIONS

 ## INHALATION METHOD

Since steam inhalation is too harsh for asthmatics, regular inhalation from the essential oil bottle or a water room diffuser will work more gently. Peppermint, Chamomile, Lemon, Mandarin, Cypress, Frankincense and Eucalyptus Radiata are more soothing for asthma sufferers when used in this way.

 ## ASTHMA CHEST RUB

A chest rub is my favorite for this condition. A great blend is eight drops of Cypress, three drops of Peppermint and five drops of Frankincense mixed with one tablespoon of vegetable oil. Massage this mixture over your chest and apply a warm compress for five minutes.

 ## BRONCHITIS

Our lungs are among the body's largest organs. The air enters our bodies through the windpipe (trachea) and connects with the bronchi, our breathing tubes that lead into the alveoli, the air sacs in the lungs. Then the exchange with carbon dioxide happens. When you have bronchitis, you suffer from an inflammation in the bronchial tubes. You have mucus build-up, coughing, chest and back pain, sore throat, fever, chills and shivering. You are officially a mess! When you have acute bronchitis, it is caused by an infection (bacterial or viral), usually after you have been sick with a cold or influenza. If left untreated, you can develop pneumonia. Chronic bronchitis is caused by frequent irritation of the lungs due to exposure to cigarette smoke, pollutants and toxic fumes.

When something is too toxic for me, I usually huff and puff like and old car that did not pass its annual smog test. My nose is my radar and my lungs are my best barometers for a health hazard. I am extra sensitive to synthetic perfumes and pollutants. When you inhale pure natural essential oils, you are providing your body with a natural cleansing experience that improves your oxygen intake and boosts your immunity. Always travel with my aromatherapy box.

 ## SOLUTIONS

 ## INHALATION METHOD FOR BRONCHITIS

From the bottle, just inhale gently one of these single oils one after the other, like a rainbow. Basil, Cypress, Ginger, Sandalwood, Ginger, Thyme, Eucalyptus, Pine, Lavender, Lemon, Mandarin, Frankincense and finally, Tea Tree oil.

 ## CHEST RUB for Bronchitis

 ## BREATH BOOSTER:

Five drops of Eucalyptus (*Eucalyptus globulus*), a great expectorant and decongestant, antibacterial, antiseptic and analgesic agent.

Eight drops of Tea Tree oil (*Melaleuca alternifolia*), it has powerful antifungal and antibacterial properties, and is amazing for respiratory disorders.

Eight drops of Pine (*Pinus sylvestris*), it is an excellent expectorant—superb for cleaning the phlegm from your lungs. It has a masculine balsamic aroma. It is "<u>tha bomb!</u>" Mix these babies in a 10 ml solution of carrier oil, apply on the chest and cover with a warm compress for five minutes.

 ## SINUSITIS

Sometimes after a cold, flu or hay fever crisis, your drainage system, AKA sinuses, go on strike and a bacterial infection sets in. Then you feel the pressure in the sinuses and the head, and the headaches can be quite intense. The congestion can become so bad that you cannot breathe through your nose, only through your mouth. You have sinusitis.

 ## INHALATION

Mix together five drops of Eucalyptus, five drops of Peppermint and three drops of Lemon. Sniff sniff sniff. I <u>love</u> that blend. Simple and gentle, but laser beam focused on reopening your sinuses.

I also like Lavender, Pine, Ginger, Frankincense and Thyme for a single oil inhalation method.

 ## EMERGENCY CASE STUDY WITH BRONCHITIS IN FRANCE

Years ago in Europe, I met with one of my very best friends from Norway. She has a beautiful 17th century French villa in France, la Marmande, Saint-Pierre-sur-Dropt, in the Southwest of France near Bordeaux. Tone had been sick with cold and flu, then laryngitis and bronchitis for over a month. She just flew in from Norway and once at "Le Bardeche," her family villa, she collapsed in bed with no more juice or voice. I looked at her mother Wenche (an ex nurse and breast cancer survivor who I affectionately call my Norwegian Mother), and we both hightailed it into their medieval kitchen to cook up a great remedy. I crushed garlic gloves, onions, cayenne pepper and cloves together with lemon juice and olive oil. Then I mixed that poultice with one drop each of these essential oils: Lemon, Lavender, Thyme, Pine, Peppermint, Clove, Cinnamon, Tea Tree, Basil, Eucalyptus, and, finally, Ginger.

Wow, the smell was intense! I applied it on her chest with a towel and a plastic bag to keep the poultice from evaporating. I also applied it under her feet with big woolen socks, then I covered them with plastic bags on each foot to make sure the poultice would hold on to her body during the night. She slept very late the next morning, and then she walked into the kitchen and spoke to us with her normal voice and a rested face. Thanks to some fresh produce and herbs, and, of course, my apothecary aroma box that I always carry with me when I travel, she was not sick any more. Yippie! She said she could taste all the food and natural remedies in her mouth when she woke up that morning.

 MARINA'S TRAVEL KIT

My travel kit contains the basic oils needed for travel and for common illnesses while traveling, including upset stomach, colds and headaches... I am listing these again for your convenience.

 MARINA MERMAID FIRST AID and TRAVEL KIT

Clove (*Syzygium aromaticum*), Eucalyptus (*Eucalyptus Globulus*), German Chamomile (*Matricaria chamomilla*), Geranium

(*Pelargonium graveolens*), Ginger (*Zingiber Officinalis*), Grapefruit (*Citrus x Paradisi*), Lavender (*Lavandula angustifolia*), Lemon (*Citrus limonum*), Lemongrass (*Cymbopogon citratus*), Patchouli (*Pogostemon patchouli*), Peppermint (*Mentha piperita*), Tea Tree (*Melaleuca alternifolia*), Thyme (*Thymus vulgaris*)

These 13 essential oils are my favorite single oils to carry.

I carry much more than this because I like choices, options and great smells. But this list is really fantastic to have because it will cover a larger umbrella of ailments such as cuts, burns, insomnia, sunburn, jetlag, fever, cramps, blisters, food poisoning, questionable or smelly bedding, travel sickness, swelling, rashes, infections, sprains, sunstroke, wounds, bed bugs and insect bites.

*Women need real moments of
solitude and self-reflection to balance
out how much of ourselves
we give away.*
-Barbara de Angelis

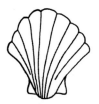

Seashell #8
Calm Down Your Raging Hormones—the Solution to PMS, Hot Flashes, Stretch Marks and More so You Can Reclaim the Sexy Goddess You Are

In Quebec, when someone is overreacting to a situation we would say: "Relax your hormones," (*Relaxes-toi les hormones!*). Hormones are sometimes the cause of many "situations" created between people—sometimes not so funny, sometimes not so cool. I am talking here about PMS, pre-menstrual syndrome. In this crucial seashell I want to talk about PMS, dysmenorrhea (difficult periods), menopause and hot flashes, breast awareness, libido and sex appeal.

Premenstrual syndrome can be like your family members arriving at your house unannounced. You would rather be ready for them and organized with enough food, clean sheets and planned activities. PMS can arrive whenever it feels like it—these physical symptoms can start to happen from the moment you ovulate in mid-cycle until you menstruate.

When what we used to call "Liberal Aunty" arrives, the PMS roller coaster stops. Ahhhhh. What can alleviate this pre-period aggravation? Geranium essential oil is the key. If you feel tired, Geranium is known as a great adrenal booster. The adrenal cortex is where your estrogens and androgens (for males) are produced, and these hormones are very important to help you feel balanced. It is vital to include Geranium essential oil to help with any menstrual disorders. PMS can make you violent and aggressive, weepy and depressed, irritable and very tired. If you feel that any of these symptoms describe you at "that time of the month," please do yourself a big favor and make yourself a potent belly oil in advance to take care of yourself when you get the monthly "visitor."

 ## PMS BLENDS

 ### *Dragon Lady Flush* BELLY OIL

Geranium, Grapefruit, Rose with Evening Primrose carrier oil.

Simply massage your belly a few days before your period with a blend of Evening Primrose (*Oenothera biennis*), a beautiful carrier oil with anti-inflammatory therapeutic properties. This is your best friend for PMS and regulation of your menstrual cycle. It is full of GLA (gamma linoleic acid), minerals and vitamins. I love mixing a tablespoon of Evening Primrose with five drops of Geranium (*Pelargonium graveolens*) to help with mood swings, ten drops of Grapefruit (*Citrus x paradisi*) to give you more energy and relieve your pre-menstrual tension and five drops of Rose (*Bulgar* or *Maroc*) to help you if you are super sad and you need to be more balanced. It is also great tonic for your uterus. This blend is a nice way to put your "Dragon Lady" on the leash.

In aromatherapy school, I experimented a lot with the oils. When I applied a little Geranium oil on my belly, instead of having a period for three days, it would cut it to a day and a half.

I recommend starting with just one application, adjusting as needed for the heaviness of your flow. For some women this blend is very strong, so only one belly rub will be necessary. Missing your period completely or spotting is to be avoided; you just want to lessen the flow. Once you get the rhythm of how your body wants to menstruate, go ahead and massage your belly morning and night for the amount of days that's right for you before your period. If you forget to use it just before your period, and apply it during your period instead, it will take a bit longer for your symptoms to quiet down.

When I rub it on the bellies of my clients, they calm down and the spasms and pain stop in about five minutes.

The quantity of oils used can be extended by making a spritzer. It's easy to make the blends beforehand and then put the mixture into a spritzer bottle found in a drugstore, pharmacy or apothecary. You can also order these sleek spritzers from my company along with your oils. This is a great way to ensure that you are not distracted by pain at work, when you're out and about or traveling.

Below are recipes for blends of easy-to-use portable spritzers to ease PMS discomfort no matter where you might be.

❀ *Pump the Peace* blend and spritzer for stress and irritability.

Frankincense, Sweet Orange, Ylang Ylang, with Apricot Kernel carrier oil.

For spritzer, just mix ten drops of the blend in 10 ml of water. Spritz it over your head and enjoy.

🌸 **Pump the Joy** blend and spritzer for depression/sadness Bergamot, Jasmine sambac absolute, Neroli, Peppermint, Rose Otto with Apricot Kernel carrier oil. For Spritzer, use ten drops of the blend in 10 ml of water. Spritz over your head and enjoy.

When you spritz, you get the benefit of oils from inhalation in a spritzer, and you can stretch your single oils and blends for many, many months. I say, "Extend the blend!"

🐚 SINGLE OIL REMEDY FOR CRAMPS

I was at the airport going through customs in Seattle and I started having the most horrendous cramps I've ever had in my life. Thank goodness I had my trusty bottle of Peppermint oil in my purse. I quickly put five drops of Peppermint on my belly, and by the time I reached the lineup at customs, the cramps had stopped. Peppermint is an anti-spasmodic. When I got to the car, I simply massaged my belly for five minutes. This is a natural way to relieve the pain of menstruation.

For at-home use, I would recommend ten drops of Peppermint in an emergency, for sudden onset of gut-ripping cramps.

🌸 **Dragon Lady Flush Dysmenorrhea** PERIOD BLEND

Do you suffer from painful and difficult periods? So painful that you cannot go to work or to school? Forty percent of women suffer form PMS and two thirds of women are afflicted by dysmenorrhea. The worst is the heavy bleeding. So for you, my sisters, the hot bottle on the belly is always a blissful relief for sure. To stop the cramps as well you need an antispasmodic blend.

Here comes 🌸 *Dragon Lady Flush for Dysmenorrhea*

Lemon, Geranium, Peppermint in evening primrose carrier oil.

Just massage your Evening Primrose on your belly (one tablespoon) with eight drops of Peppermint (*Mentha piperita*). To stop the cramps and cool you down, add five drops of Lemon (*Citrus limonum*) for tension release, and finally five drops of Geranium (*Pelargonium graveolens*) to help stop your bleeding and regulate your menstrual flow, like a reliable traffic controller keeping you safe. Every time I use this blend I notice I have a shorter period and the cramps are under control really quickly because of the hemostatic property of Geranium oil, which cuts bleeding. I enjoy applying a warm compress on my abdomen for ten minutes to make the cramps stop. This is a relaxing way to heal your belly when your periods are out of control.

The idea behind a spritzing experience or an aromatherapy massage is all about self-nurturing during this time of the month. I enjoyed John Gray's new book 🌟 *Why Mars and Venus Collide*. He discusses the importance of women nurturing themselves. He explains that the hormone oxytocin (from the Greek meaning sweet birth), the hormone of love and cuddling, is massively produced for women during a massage. When the woman feels heard and safe, she relaxes. The benefit of spritzing yourself with essential oils is the comforting reminder of the caring massage you had the month before.

🐚 MENOPAUSE

Menopause, simply put, means you are running out of eggs and are completing the fertile time of your life. It can take some women many years to finally reach the completion of their menstrual cycle. You heard about some women getting pregnant at 60 years old? Really, it can be such a vast span.

Some women start menopause in their thirties or it can indeed take until the late fifties or even sixties until the egg production finally stops. Symptoms can range from headaches to hot flashes, dry skin, dryness of the vagina and an inability to focus. There are an abundance of essential oils that you can use to gain relief from these symptoms.

 ## MENOPAUSE RELIEF BLENDS

❧ *Headache Gooone*

Spritzer

Lavender, Spearmint and Peppermint essential oils mixed with Apricot Kernel carrier oil.

Use ten drops of the blend in ten ml of water. Spritz and sniff.

❧ *Flow*

Body oil/perfume

Evening Primrose, Rosehip carrier oil, Sunflower carrier oil, Jojoba and Camellia and Geranium essential oils.

Massage ❧ *Flow* on your neck/thyroid gland area, your abdomen and your face before bedtime. This blend helps you transcend sluggishness and boosts low energy levels, especially if you have hypo thyroid. It is also great for mature skin and smoothing fine lines.

 ## HOT FLASHES

When your blood vessels are irregular in their function, causing a yo-yo effect of constricting and dilating, you enter the spinning world of hot flashes. Your blood flow increases, raising your body temperature and also increasing your heart rate. You suddenly become as red as a tomato in a middle of a conversation and then you're wiping your brow as you break into a sweat. Sound familiar?

The ❀ *Dragon Lady Flush Hot Flash Blend* and spritzer will refresh and cool you down.

The best carrier oil is our champion Evening Primrose. Massage one tablespoon of it on your belly combined with five drops of Geranium, five drops Lemon and five drops of Grapefruit essential oils. You can use ten drops of this blend in a spritzer bottle with water. Shake it and spritz it over your head and face when you are having a hot flash/sweat episode.

❀ *Dragon Lady Flush Hot Flash Blend*

A 10 ml oil blend.

❀ *Dragon Lady Flush Hot Flash Spritzer*

In 10 ml of water, add ten drops of your Dragon Lady Flush Hot Flash blend. Shake and spritz.

Go ahead, you've earned it. Take the spritzer right out of your purse and spritz yourself right there in the restaurant. There, don't you feel better?

Great for mature skin!

❀ *Chillax Blend for Anxiety*

Frankincense, Sweet Orange, Jasmine in 10 ml of Jojoba oil blend. This is one of my clients' favorite blends/spritzers when they need to let go.

❀ *Chillax Spritzer*, use ten drops of the blend in our 10 ml water spritzer. Helps you chill and relax so you can ride comfortably through the rollercoaster of your symptoms.

BREAST AWARENESS

The "Milkshake" song by Kelis, with its chorus "my milkshake brings the boys in the yard," makes me laugh so much. Ode to the girls! How are your girls these days? I love my breasts, 100% natural (no implants) I care for them a lot.

I have been labeled a voluptuous, breasty girl most of my life. I remember when they appeared in puberty like a Christmas Gift dropped from the sky from Santa. I was aware of being noticed more and more... by men, if you know what I mean.

I worked in our family business as young as 13 years old as a cashier and gas girl. That's my sister and me on "Gas Girls un monde en folie" on YouTube. We were on a TV show in 1982, someone later found the footage and put it up on YouTube, and it's had more than 8,000 hits. Travelers would come to our tiny town and ask, "Where are the Gas Girls? I want to see the Gas Girls!"

I was pumping gas throughout my teenager years. I think it helped me to be less shy with men in general. When you grow up in a garage surrounded by testosterone, you have to learn to establish your space with your gifted bundle of estrogen. Many women slouch and hide their breasts.

For me, breast awareness started when I felt how heavy my breasts were. I made sure I cherished them and carried them in a proper harness. My favorite gear is the ✗ Tab Bra from www.tabbra.com, designed by Yvonne. This bra offers optimal support and posture correction for better circulation. I learned over the years that underwire bras suffocate the lymph nodes that are right under the breasts, and it is much better to get the full suspension from your shoulders with larger straps.

When I exercise, I like to wear full suspension. My girlfriend Tami (my personal icon for image solutions) told me once that only wearing the sports bra gave me the uniboob look. She said that I had to split the girls by wearing a lifting bra under the sports bra. She was right. Now I feel better and more supported. Trying to run with a bad bra is painful! I also make sure I do not wear any bra when I am at home. I set my girls on the loose.

It is very healthy to nurture your breasts—they are the extension of your heart chakra, your love center and also the self-nurturing mezzanine (balcony) in your body. When you nurture your precious feminine assets, you are paying attention to your heart area, opening your heart. Treating yourself with love enables you to nurture others with peacefulness, without feelings of resentment or sacrifice.

I enjoyed working with Diane with aromatherapy and reflexology, the feet are the gates of your soul and I am very delighted for Diane's discovery.

"Marina, I took away from our session two things that stuck with me. The first is the amazing association between the feet and the other locations in your body. The reflexology. I was very relaxed. The essential oils you used during the massage were also very soothing for me.

The second and most memorable was when you told me to make sure that we each love ourselves. It sounds like common sense. This really helped me. I tell my boys five to seven times a day that I love them. I have always done this. I also tell my husband and my mom that I love them. I never thought about loving myself. I am always hard on myself and strive for perfection in certain aspects of my life. My oldest son, Markus, who is ten, is similar. I have thought about loving myself since this conversation and it has helped. I thank you for this. Every time I inhale the essential oils I bought from you I remember to love myself."

Diane Rauch

Mom and Contract Worker

Abbotsford, B.C.

CASTOR OIL BREAST TREATMENT

For a deep breast cleansing poultice use castor oil on a 100% piece of cotton and apply it to your breasts. Relax for half and hour. This is a folk remedy that is super-powerful for removing toxins.

The essentials oils are my best friends. I have a history of cystic breasts, and to help to reduce the lumps that come and go, I mix evening primrose carrier oil (two tablespoons) with Cypress (eight drops), Chamomile (eight drops) and Lavender (eight drops) and massage my breasts as often I can with this mix. It keeps the cysts down.

Years ago, I had the chance to receive aromatherapy treatments combined with the Derma Ray Technology. I had a huge lump in my left breast and after five sessions with this system, the lump decreased by 80%. I was so happy about that, I decided to become an aromatherapist so I could get my training to use the Derma Ray unit in my practice. I studied with Dr. Sabina M. De Vita at the DeVita Wellness Institute of Living and Learning in Ontario.

Dr. DeVita is an amazing teacher and she is also the author of ✴ *Electromagnetic Pollution*. I have been using the Derma Ray Technology quite a bit in the last five years. As I mentioned earlier, it helps to move the lymph in the body, reduce the size of your fat cells, stimulate your circulation and leaves you feeling light and fresh. I also make sure to receive an aromatherapy massage every four weeks.

The triangle of balance for me is good food and nutrition, good rest and relaxation, good fun and playtime. I also enjoy natural products on my skin. My lymph nodes, located in my armpit area (called axillary nodes), are never treated with any antisudorifics, i.e. antiperspirants, because they contain aluminum. I do not cook with aluminum pots and pans. The pores under the arms need to breathe and I use deodorant made with essentials oils.

Cedarwood, Geranium, Lavender, Cypress, Patchouli, Pine, Sandalwood, Tea Tree, Ylang Ylang, Eucalyptus, Clary Sage, and Bergamot can be used to great effect singly as your armpit refresher. Use a spray bottle or a roll-on bottle and mix them with water, apple cider vinegar (excellent to maintain your skin PH level) or crystal mist deodorant. This liquefied crystal is also a great base to mix your essential oils with. Crystal mist liquid deodorant is usually imported from Thailand and it is a miracle natural deodorant made of mineral salts called potassium alum, also known simply as alum or less simply, potassium aluminum sulfate dodecahydrate. Although it has aluminum in the name, it is considered a paraben, which is propylene glycol and aluminum free. It is usually mixed with purified water and the essential oils of your choice.

But my favorite natural deodorant recipe is:

Mix 20 drops each of Pine, Sandalwood and Patchouli in a 50 ml bottle of your favorite carrier (water and apple cider vinegar or crystal mist liquid). This natural deodorant is a dream in a bottle!

 ## PREGNANT GODDESS

If you are pregnant and are looking for a great way to keep your belly skin smooth and silky, mix ten drops of Neroli oil, ten drops of Lavender, and ten drops of Mandarin in a 50 ml bottle of avocado oil or Apricot Kernel or Sweet Almond carrier oil and massage every day to prevent stretch marks.

All my friends who were pregnant used it, and they got their husbands to massage it in for them. Each and every one of them reported that they didn't have any stretch marks.

 ## BREASTFEEDING

Breastfeeding is so good for your baby, and to make sure you produce enough of your precious milk, massage one drop of Fennel, one drop of Geranium and one drop of Lemongrass in one tablespoon of vegetable oil on your breasts and apply a warm compress for ten minutes. It will stimulate your milk production, a galactogogue effect.

At the end of your breastfeeding cycle as a mother, use three drops of Peppermint and massage your breasts with it, then apply a warm compress for ten minutes. Peppermint will help to stop your milk production, an antigalactogogic effect.

Breast Tissue Toning Oil is great for giving your breasts the firmness they deserve. Mix three drops of Lemongrass, three drops of Geranium together with three drops of Carrot Seed oil (*Daucus carota*), which is so wonderful for skin care, into two tablespoons of vegetable oil. Apply it on your breasts after your morning shower.

Breast tissue soothing oil is essential when your breasts are sore. Mix three drops of Geranium with three drops of Lavender with three drops of Carrot Seed (*Daucus carota*) essential oil in two tablespoons of vegetable oil. Massage gently over the breasts when they are tender.

 ## BREAST CANCER NOTE

Breast cancer took my grand-maman Yvette and my Aunty Suzanne away. My dear stepmom (more like a sister to me) Huguette, is a gracious survivor in our family. My father would tell us kids: *"Depechons-nous d'etre heureux"* ("Let's hurry up and be happy!").

I want to honor all the women who are confronting breast cancer. They are our teachers in our quest to nurture ourselves into health. All my life I have been encouraging people around me to adopt a healthy lifestyle with increased exercise, weight control and improved nutrition. Those are major lifestyle changes that you can make one step at a time to have powerful effects on reducing your risk.

My best recommendation regarding cancer and essential oils is to invite into your world the <u>inhalation</u> of oils that make you feel better. Please use the oils to elevate your mood during this time of sickness. From experience with friends, family and clients afflicted with cancer, the citrus family is always a great way to uplift your spirits: Grapefruit, Orange, Lemon, Lime and Mandarin.

 ## LET'S TALK ABOUT SEX, BABY (AND ESSENTIAL OILS)

Now let's talk about your vibrations regarding your sex life. You can expand your "After Sex Glow vibrations" with these eight easy fresh 🕊 wings 🕊.

Have you noticed how much more attractive you feel after you had really <u>great sex</u>?

Are you "turned on" by yourself? If you are not, there is a good chance your potential partner will not be either.

Your nose knows… when you feel a magnetic pull toward someone, there is sexual attraction. The power of pheromones is very exciting to say the least. From Wikipedia, the word pheromone comes from the Greek *phero* "to bear" and *hormone* "impetus," or driving force.

A pheromone is a secreted or excreted chemical factor that triggers a social response in members of the same species. Pheromones are chemicals capable of acting outside the body of the secreting individual to impact the behavior of the receiving individual. There are alarm pheromones, food trail pheromones, sex pheromones, and many others that affect behavior or physiology. When you're hungry you smell the prey, just as a fox smells a chicken in the barnyard and snatches it.

Women who produce higher-than-average amounts of female pheromones called copulins have greater success with men—success in the attraction zone. When your level of copulin and androstenol is high, you can increase the level of testosterone of a man by 150%. Then you are guaranteed pleasure.

I love blending aphrodisiacs to keep you on the <u>edge</u>. When you wear a magnificent blend of pure essential oils… watch out, this is your social lubricator, your ice-breaker, your sexual attractant. I have created this very sexy aphrodisiac for you called ❀ **Wanted**. Are you wanted? If not, wear this and see the line forming behind your buttocks. ❀ **Wanted** is described in Wing #8. Can you wait?

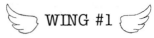

WING #1

SMILE LIKE YOU WANT TO SUNTAN YOUR TEETH. BIG SMILE!

The power of a smile is the ultimate way to connect with others and attract good energy into your life. If you have a "concrete face"—you are super-serious all the time and afraid to smile because you may break your stony face—please try it. Remember, it takes 17 muscles to smile and 47 muscles to frown. When you smile you say yes to life, to people, to the universe, to love. Smile like you want to suntan your teeth. It will raise your vibrations big time.

To help you to smile better, you can use my lip balm 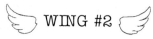 *Lick & Bite* with beeswax and maple syrup from my Dad's sugar shack in Quebec. Your lips will be sexy-smooth and hydrated. Mmmouah, sweet kisses. XXX

🪽 WING #2 🪽

GLOWING SKIN

Your skin needs attention and scrubbing with the **Renaissance Glove** is step number one when you shower. Using essential oils to heal yourself includes using body lotions with essential oils. The added benefit is that they will make you feel like a luxurious princess. Make sure your temple is strong by exercising to keep your body solid as a rock. A firm body is a precious asset for your health. Build up that muscle tone to protect your bones.

To help you to feel hydrated use the all-natural silky skin lotions I carry: 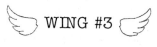 *Marie-Jeanne de France* (Lavender); *Creamsicle* (Mandarin and Vanilla); *After Sex Glow* (Ylang Ylang); *Aloha Mermaid* (Kukui oil from Hawaii and Gardenia/Plumeria); *Buddha Yoga Fresh* (Lemongrass); *Gladiator Awakening* (Peppermint/ Spearmint). Gel soaps are also available.

🪽 WING #3 🪽

 GROUNDING MEDITATION

Step into the vortex of creation by starting to relax and meditate a few minutes per day. Visualize the opening between

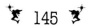

you and the Divine, Source, God, Goddess, your vertical alignment with your Higher Self and the Source of all things. Stop resisting your gift and surrender to be able to share your blessings. Living in creative ecstasy is my dream life and I am the creator of my life.

Surround yourself with essential oils to help you connect with and live in your full creatorship. Make sure you have a spiritual sanctuary in your home, in your room, in your car, in the forest, at work… whatever does it for you. I tremendously enjoy ✳ Snatam Kaur's Sanskrit songs for that. Music is such a pleasant way to elevate your spiritual connection with the Infinite. As above, so below, the infinity sideways 8 shape is a great symbol to use as well. These products will help you get into a meditation or a clear and peaceful zone:

❀ *Salute the Sun* spritzer (water, Neroli, Jasmine, Lemon)

❀ *Green Wing* spritzer (water, Cypress, Peppermint, Lime)

❀ *White Wing* spritzer (water, Lavender, Orange, Sandalwood)

NOSE JOB INHALERS: ❀ *Crystal Clear,* ❀ *Sports,* ❀ *I Believe,* ❀ *Pure Potential,* ❀ *Limitless* to help you to stimulate your right brain so you activate your pure creative inspiration with a grounding foundation. Remember your nose knows what you need. Trust your instinct to pick the right one for you.

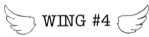 WING #4

POWER OF YOUR LEFT HAND AND TANTRIC SEX

Can you hear the famous sensual song of Marvin Gaye, "Sexual Healing" now?

My left hand is my best friend. Never disappointed by her, she knows what to do to please me unconditionally. Libido is in the head, the heart, the body. Libido is like a savage wild horse, it comes and it goes. Libido lives in the fantasia world of your imagination. I enjoy riding the waves of my libido. When I am horny and frisky, I know I am still _alive_ and the flow of my sexual energy is guiding me to the ultimate paroxysm of an orgasmic rollercoaster that only I know how to enjoy. Ode to the left hand, which can be your best friend. Tantric sex is also a pure gateway to the best connection of intense sexual and spiritual experience between two souls.

"Sexual energy is one of our most powerful energies for creating health," says Christiane Northrup, M.D., author of _Women's Bodies, Women's Wisdom._ By using our sexual energy consciously, we can tap into a true source of youth and vitality.

Tantra emerged in India more than 6,000 years ago. Tantra sprang up as a rebellion against organized religion, which held that sexuality should be rejected in order to reach enlightenment. Sexuality is our doorway to the divine. Earthly pleasures such as eating, dancing and creative expression are sacred acts. The word Tantra means "to manifest, to expand, to show and to weave." In this context, sex is the expansion of our consciousness and weaves together the polarities of male (Shiva, Hindu God) and female (Shakti, Hindu Goddess) into a harmonious whole. Tantric practices teach us to prolong the act of making love and how to utilize potent orgasmic energies more effectively.

Are you afraid, fascinated, curious, aroused by your sexuality? Listen to your internal compass and open the door.

Massage yourself and your partner with this blend. To help

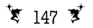

you relax and connect, please enjoy ✿ *Sexy Mermaid Body Oil* of Evening Primrose, Apricot Kernel, Jojoba, Vitamin E and Ylang Ylang (*Cananga odorata*) to help your odyssey and voyage through sensuality.

🦋 WING #5 🦋

MINDSET SHIFT

You really want to be in the "cool girl, cool woman" category. Why? Because when you are a cool girl, it is because you are in charge of your emotions, you have a great attitude and people want to be in your company because they enjoy being with you. Mindset is so vital. When you believe in yourself and your dreams, your world is rock on. If you do not believe in yourself, it is hard for people to believe in you.

The mindset is top priority. Your beliefs are working for and with you when you attract successful relationships and situations in your life. Your thoughts will create your emotions and will propel you to take action. Are you an action-taker? Are you walking the talk? Are you eager to succeed?

I always enjoy connecting with ordinary people who are accomplishing extraordinary things. Life is so short, dive in and live. With my Equinox circle sister EM from Colorado, we use this mantra, *"I am stepping into my power, setting boundaries, speaking my authentic truth every day effortlessly."* And then we laugh at all the miracles and synchronicities that happen to us. Marvelous!

The ✿ *Nose Job* inhaler called ✿ *I Believe* is highly recommended to make sure you will stop talking about it and start doing it!

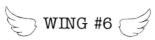

WING #6

POWER OF DRESSING UP

I really enjoy the before-and-after story of an ordinary-looking person who is suddenly transformed in an "extreme makeover" experience. With the help of a team of experts, from head to toe, this person is catapulted to another level of success and their ultimate potential.

I am always so excited to see the change and the reactions of the entourage surrounding this Cinderella. They do not believe it is the same person. After losing the extra weight, getting the right haircut and the best style of clothes for their body, the teeth are done, the skin is treated, and the experts, life coach, fitness trainer, stylists are all there to support the transformation process. This butterfly is born with the help of this team of experts. Lovely. It's the ultimate TV show to watch and produces a fabulous, strong message of hope for the chosen one. The power of stepping up is huge in our society right now and Marie-Lyne and I are working on this cocoon that we call *Wings of Transformation* (*Les Elles de la Transformation*), to help you to metamorphose with a solid team of experts. Stay tuned.

Learn how to dress to attract, dress to seduce, dress to relax (in French *"on s'habille en mou"* means wearing soft and comfy clothes to relax). I am not the best for fashion, but I enjoy getting help from image-makers who have the eagle eye to help maximize the look for each body type. Seek help if you need it so you can accentuate your assets and feel good in your clothes.

For years I used to hide my breasts. Now I honor my female energy by wearing a more open concept for "the girls," if you know what I mean. I was just shy that way.

To help your self-esteem to soar, enjoy the ❀ *Nose Job* inhaler called ❀ *Pure Potential*. Be free and be you.

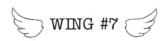

POWER OF THE HIPS

Move your hips. Shakira's song "Give It Up to Me" makes me want to move my hips on and on and on. You can have it all, anything you want in the world! What a sexy mermaid is this Latina Shakira.

I have been fascinated with water, waves, mermaids and frogs since I was a little girl. The frog is the symbol for cleansing and detox is the water element. I am also French Canadian, a _frog_! I _love_ dance, dancing, and watching people dance. I love movement, wave motions. My hips are my barometer for my joy factor. When I am happy, my hips are rolling a lot, red carpet walk, model walk and all, bring it on baby! It makes me laugh so hard!

When I came to Vancouver for a quick (one month) pop in 1995, I saw the Little Mermaid on her Rock. You can see her in Stanley Park in Vancouver when you walk on the sea wall. I was deeply touched by her. I followed my heart and traveled to the West Coast, finally.

I also fell in love with the statue of the Angel of Victory helping a fallen soldier to ascend. This iconic bronze statue in Gastown was designed by Coeur de Lion McCarthy in 1921 in remembrance of the 1100 Canadian Pacific Railway workers who died in WWI and WWII. It has a very Renaissance vibe for me. When I arrived in Vancouver in August of 1997, I climbed the statue and held the hand of that soldier too. My soldier of Love. This is one of my favorite pictures of Vancouver. No wonder why my Marina Mermaid logo is an angel and a mermaid holding a pearl high in the sky.

The legends of mermaids are infinite. I like the one telling the story of a mermaid sitting on a rock while combing her long hair with her comb made of seashell. She manifested two human legs and hid her mermaid skin tail under the rock. Mermaids enjoy celebrations with dancing and singing. Mermaids love dancing, and dancing with humans. They can fall in love effortlessly at first sight. They can make a man fall in love with them too. Sometimes, they get played by a man who knows the legend of hiding the mermaid's tail so that she can never return home to the sea.

I heard many times from fitness experts that the hip joints are made to move and when your hip joints are flowing and full of synovial liquid, your life is flowing and your health is vibrant. Moving forward by keeping your hips flexible is a powerful way of growing in wisdom and keeping your youth factor. When you dance, just go fishing in your "spank bank" to connect your vibes with your sexy energy.

Move your hips as much as you can. Belly dancing is an excellent way to connect with your Eros fire. Your yin female energy is flourishing the most when you learn a new way to shake your booty. Hip hop is cool to me cause it feels very yang/masculine energy and the yin and yang are blending very smoothly when I hip hop dance.

Promise yourself you will learn a new style: Latin dance, line dance with your cowboy hat and sexy boots, whatever makes you laugh. Know that your second chakra (wheel of energy in Sanskrit), which is located in your abdomen, lower back and sexual organs, is all about your sexual energy and how you feel your emotions. Let's dance! You can massage your belly with a few drops of ❀ *Flow* and ❀ *Sexy Mermaid* so you can ignite yourself to dance like nobody's watching!

❀ *Flow* organic body oil/perfume is made with evening primrose oil, which is an excellent anti-inflammatory that also helps to stabilize cholesterol problems. Apricot Kernel oil is also an excellent anti-inflammatory oil loaded with vitamins A, D and E. Jojoba oil, our natural preservative oil, is also an anti-inflammatory. The Geranium essential oil (*Pelargonium graveolens*) is great for activation of your lymph and circulation. ❀ *Flow* can help you move your body and feel confident in your body. It can be used as a natural perfume.

❀ *Sexy Mermaid* organic body oil/perfume is made with the same anti-inflammatory carrier oils of Evening Primrose, Apricot Kernel, Jojoba and Ylang Ylang (*Cananga odorata*) essential oil for calming you down if you are in a panic mode. It is also excellent for female reproductive problems. The smell is super sweet and many admirers feel smitten when they get a whiff of this oil.

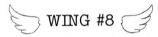

WING #8

BE TURNED ON BY YOURSELF

Remember that song "I'm Too Sexy" by the artist Right Said Fred? "I'm too sexy for my shirt…"

Being a woman has many powerful advantages. When you step into your power and express your sexual vibes, your sex appeal becomes mesmerizing, and your X Factor propels you through the roof. You are in charge of launching love arrows. I call it "sending out circles," like a stone thrown into a pond. You are channeling higher frequencies like a radio station that everybody wants to listen to. Your antennas are buzzing. Make sure you know how hot you are. Do you feel hot and burning, beautiful and gorgelicious? Because when you step into this powerful state of the burning flame of the female matrix, you make people feel better, more loved and more peaceful around you. You can always turn up the wattage of your charming quantity of attributes to maintain high vibrations of love in your life. Honor it!

To help you to feel hotter, enjoy the aphrodisiac *Wanted*, made of Jojoba oil with Jasmine, Patchouli, Orange, Grapefruit, Sandalwood, Frankincense, Ylang Ylang, Black Pepper and <u>love</u>. Tap into your Aphrodite Greek Goddess of love and enjoy the ride. You deserve it! I really enjoy working with women that are empowered by self-nurturing experiences. Heather is a senior firefighter who knows how to attract women into indulgence, fun and relaxation. She is the Wonder Woman I know in real life! I'm relaxing the world one woman at a time!

Marina's services have been a part of Ultimate Scrapbook Retreats for over five years. From the over 500 women that attend our retreats, Marina has probably treated most of them at least once and many of them several times. Marina has won the hearts of all the ladies that attend our retreats with her caring and genuinely friendly and welcoming personality. The attendees have come to expect Marina to be there and have grown to love her!

With the wide range of services she offers, everything from angel card readings, ear candling to aromatherapy massages and reflexology... She is a very busy lady at our retreats. Every client comes away happy and re-energized!

For myself, as the organizer, Marina has been great to work with. Her attention to detail and professionalism along with her easy-going attitude helps make an appointment with Marina unforgettable.

Our retreats would not be the same without Marina's awesome smile and positive energy!

Heather Wilson

Ultimate Scrapbook Retreats Organizer and Burnaby Senior Firefighter

British Columbia, Canada

www.ultimatescrapbookretreats.blogspot.com

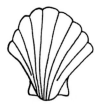

Children's Seashell
Kids and Essential Oils

Children are precious and they are sensitive. I wish I had known an aromatherapist when I was a child. I know now that the power of smell is very important. I am very fond of essential oils used in a diffuser for kids. It has to be gentle—very low dilution is best. Remember with children, <u>less is more</u>. My goal is to share the power of the essential oils with special and sensitive kids that are affected by stress, anxiety and hyperactivity.

"I am only nine years old and I feel warm, fuzzy, relaxed, safe and secure when I see Marina. A spiritual experience, I love the citrus essential oils, the lip balm with maple syrup and the sweetness of it. Cozy girl, flower and power, quality time one on one with Marina's session".

Jessica Brisdon

North Vancouver

B.C.

Coriander, Dill, Eucalyptus Citriodora, Roman Chamomile, Fir, Frankincense, Helichrysum, Lavender, Manuka, Myrtle, Neroli, Palmarosa, Petitgrain, Ravensara, Rosewood, Sandalwood, Spikenard, Tea Tree and Vetiver are very soft and sweet oils to use for diffusing with kids around the house. They also enjoy the citrus family as well.

Always keep essential oils out of young children's reach. The best time of their life for your children is when you give them one-on-one quality time. The diffuser with water and few drops of essential oils (five drops) in their rooms can begin fifteen minutes prior to bedtime so you set the tone for relaxation in their world. This is the best time to connect with them with a lovely bedtime story.

They will thank you for that.

My Maman Pierrette would sing to us before she closed our bedroom door: "Rou-dou-dou-dou-dou!"

It does not make any sense, but it meant the world when she sang it and waved her hand in a circular motion—saying ta-ta—to me as a kiddo!

Bonne Nuit! Je t'aime!

Tami, Jacqueline, Marina and Yuki
at Serenity Studio Beauty
by Jacqueline.

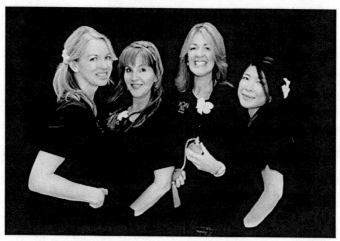

Because I am a two-time cancer survivor, I have learned to take much better care of myself. One of the way I do this is having aromatherapy massages on a regular basis. I love the smells of Lavender, Peppermint, Spearmint and Geranium.

Marina, my Aromatherapist, is so curious and excited to create and share her passion and concoctions of healing oils. A blissful and peaceful and joyful moment of massage, I wish for all to have this experience.

Love,

Jacqueline Couture-Brisdon

Owner/operator

Beauty by Jacqueline & Co

www.beautybyjacqueline.com

"Marina and I had the pleasure of working together on film sets for many years. Although we enjoyed our work we dreamed of pursuing careers in the world of beauty and wellness. During that time my mother was battling cancer, and with the aid of Marina, she found some pain relief by the use of essential oils as additional therapy. Marina soon became my official aromatherapist, making sure Mom and I would enjoy the power of the oils. I found the essential oils helped keep us unified and protected, especially during the frequent hospital visits and ups and downs.

When my mother left this world, my dream was to become a mother and a few years later I became pregnant. Again, Marina was my aromatherapist—not only for the full nine months, but also when my healthy son Trenton was born amongst the essential oils of rose, jasmine and lavender, with spa music filling the hospital room. More recently, Marina has helped me with my uterine fibroids with the hormonal blend of oils she made me to help manage the pain and potentially shrink them. She created a mixture of Evening Primrose with Grapefruit, Geranium and Lemon for me to apply on my abdomen everyday. On my scheduled day for laser surgery, I felt grounded and prepared, and in considerably less pain. God bless the essential oils! Oh and by the way, I am now living my second dream of helping women to be beautiful with my blooming aesthetics career!"

Tami Esau, Certified Aesthetician

Serenity Studio Beauty by Jacqueline

North Vancouver, B.C., Canada.

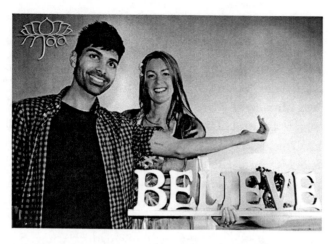

I have been a yoga teacher and studio owner for five years. Being in the wellness industry, I have been blessed to have crossed paths with so many gifted individuals, one of whom is Marina. After my first session with Marina, I felt like I had arrived home within my body; her energy and care was beyond what I had expected. She has a true gift to tap into what it is a person needs at that given moment in their life and gives a sense of peace for the mind yet a deep inner strength. I have had many moments of clarity with her and her touch is one that must be shared with others. Marina is a true healer and a very special soul. I am so honored and grateful for having the pleasure of knowing her as a friend and as a spirit healer and uplifter. Thank you—I will be eternally grateful. Life is beautiful.

Your friend,

Farhad Khan

Founder & Owner of Maa Yoga & Wellness Studio

Owner of Maa Lotus a boutique spa

Special thanks to all my dear friends in the film industry that let me touch their temples! You are Divine! Marina xxx

Amy Carlson, Bellamy Young, Bridget Moynahan, Brooke Shields, Bruce Thomas, Brittany Murphy, Chad Lowe, Chris Kramer, Christian Slater, Dhirendra, Dominic Purcell, Don Davies, Eric Stoltz, Gil Bellows, Hilary Swank, Holt McCallany, Indira Varma, Jackie Earle Haley, Jennifer Beals, Jensen Ackles, Kandice McClure, Kevin Sorbo, Kristin Lehman, Malcolm Jamal Warner, Mark Valley, Mary Steenburgen, Michelle Ryan, Mireille Enos, Molly Shannon, Nine Inch Nails (Trent Reznor), Peter O'Meara, Red Hot Chili Peppers (Anthony Kiedis), Ricky Martin crew, Robin Wright Penn, Samantha Crew, Scarlett Chorvat, Sebastien Roche, Stanley Tucci, Ted Danson, Tim Daly, Thomas Haas Chef Chocolatier, Tom Berenger, Vera Farmiga, Wesley Snipes.

A session with Marina is an experience to savour and remember. She fills your senses with the delightful aromas of her oils and strips away layers of tension with her strong and loving hands. Very relaxing and energizing.

Doug Edwards, Musician, Composer

Chilliwack band member, British Columbia

After a session with Marina and her healing hands and gentle pressure, I feel totally loved, relaxed and ready to tackle the world again. I feel so lucky and so blessed to have her in my life. XOXO

Debbie Geaghan, Costume Supervisor

Film Industry, B.C., Canada

Marina has the dedication to her craft and the personal attention to each of her clients that I look for in a wellness professional. I leave her studio feeling energized and relaxed, ready to face the stresses of the world... Til' the next time I see her anyways.

Kevin Santarossa, Prop Department,

Film Bizz, British Columbia

Marina is a genius of relaxation for your body. Her reflexology and aromatherapy massage is simply the best I have ever experienced! Her passion for health and wellness is unsurpassed.

Susie Meister

Special Events Planner, Wedding Fair

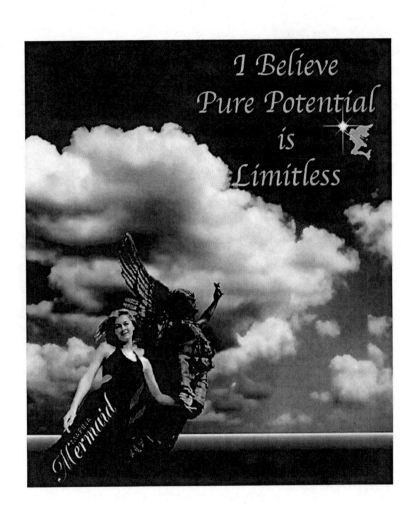

I Believe
Pure Potential
is
Limitless

APPENDIX

⟲ INHALATION PROCESS ⟳

Straight from the bottle: Open your favorite bottle and sniff with joy!

Cup your hands: Use one drop in your hands, massage hands clockwise, cup your nose and inhale.

Handkerchief or tissue: Add one drop of oil on it. You can then take the handkerchief and sniff as required, place it in the ventilation of your hotel room and blast it for ten minutes to purify the air of your room, or insert it in your pillowcase before sleep.

Steam process: Add three drops in the shower that has a steam room system and have a luxurious steamed shower. Or add two to four drops of oils to a bowl of hot water, lean your head over the bowl and inhale slowly for few minutes. Draping a towel over your head will retain the heat longer.

Diffusers for the room: Add between five and fifteen drops of oils (depending on the size of your space) in a diffuser that usually requires a good amount of water. My favorite is the ultrasonic diffuser. Follow the manufacturer's directions.

Oil burner: Add two or three drops of oils in the water on top burner heated over a candle. Follow the manufacturer's directions.

Clay Light Bulb Ring: Add two or three drops of oil on ring and place over the light bulb. Follow the manufacturer's directions.

Scent a Fire: This is amazing! Add two drops of essential oils on each log before igniting. Fabulous for Christmas!

Car diffuser: Add three drops of Peppermint, Orange or Spearmint in that electric car diffuser plugged in your lighter outlet. This will keep you alert as you drive.

Vacuum Cleaner: Place three to five drops on a cotton ball that you insert in the vacuum bag. Wonderful if you have pets.

Spritzers for Body: Add your favorite essential oils to water then shake it, spritz over your head, and inhale. Natural creamsicle: Add ten drops of Lavender and ten drops of Sweet Orange in a 60 ml spritzer bottle with spring water. This in a quick and easy thing you can do, shake it and it will create a creamsicle, a sweet comforting spritzer for you to inhale at home or at work.

Mini Spray Spritzer: Add three drops of your favorite oil or blend in this 10 ml elongated "spray spritzer" (filled with water) that has a strong pump, is refillable, sleek and compact (it looks like a cigar). Quick and easy: keep this "spray spritzer" in your purse, your car, in a drawer at work. When dealing with a negative client or boss or co-worker, simply spritz yourself off afterward.

Spritzer for Room: Add essential oils (5 ml or 100 drops) in a big bottle of 120 ml filled with water. Shake well before use, since essential oils do not dissolve in water, then spray to disinfect the room.

Hydrosol Spritzer: Use pure Lavender, pure Neroli, or pure Rose hydrosols to purify the air, over your head, on your face, on your mattress when you are changing your bedding. This is a fantastic way to purify your home with great safety.

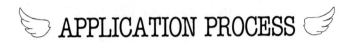

APPLICATION PROCESS

Topical application is one of the most effective means of using essential oils. According to Jean Valnet, M.D., an essential oil that is directly applied to the skin can pass into the bloodstream and diffuse throughout the tissues in 20 minutes or less.

Aromatic Bath: Add five to ten drops in water, depending on the condition, health and age of the person being treated, and depending on the oils used for detoxifying the skin, relaxing or reviving. Always pour the water first and add the oils last. It is better to mix the oils with salt or Epsom salt in the hands to dissolve everything in the water. For children, always use less, less, less!

Cold Compress: Add three to five drops in a bowl of cold water and apply the cold compress for acute inflammation such as swelling, headaches or sprains.

Hot Compress: Mix two to three drops of oil with 240 ml (one cup) of hot water and wet the washcloth, wring it out, then place on affected area until the heat dissipates. Ideal for chronic pain, muscular pain, cramps, labor.

Foot Bath: Add two to six drops of essential oil in cold or hot water, depending on the condition, health and age of the person. Soak feet for ten minutes maximum.

Hand Bath: Add two to four drops in cold or hot water, depending on the condition, health and age of the person being treated. Soak hands for five minutes maximum.

How to achieve a specific dilution: For one fluid ounce (600 drops) of carrier oil:

"Normal Dilution" is usually 2.5%, meaning 15 drops of essential oil in 1 oz of a carrier oil. Because I am often asked "How to dilute…" or "How many drops?" I have here for you these very simple dilution and measurement charts.

1% of 600   =   6 drops

2% of 600   =   12 drops

2.5% of 600   =   15 drops

5% of 600   =   30 drops

10% of 1 oz   =   60 drops

Measurements/conversions (volume)

30 ml = 1 fl oz = 600 drops = 2 tablespoons

15 ml = 1/2 oz = 300 drops = 1 tablespoon

5 ml   = 1/6 oz = 100 drops = 1 teaspoon

1 ml   = 1/30 oz = 20 drops   = 1/5 teaspoon

Massage oil for full body: The safest dilution rate for a full body massage is between 1% and 5%. If you use 2.5% for general healthy clients, you are good to go.

For clients in the higher risk category, the lower the level, the safer you are. So you can mix one or two or three drops of essential oils in 100 drops of carrier oil. If the client has a physical condition, you can increase the rate of dilution.

Massage oil for specific area: For general use, 2.5% to 5% dilution. For skin care, lower is safer, so use 0.5% to 3% dilution. For chronic physical conditions, use 5% to 10% dilution and for an acute physical condition, go with 5% to 15%. Make sure you adjust for high-risk clients.

Neat Application: One drop or two drops for an acute situation. Let's say you just burned your finger in the kitchen, one or two drops of pure Lavender on the finger will prevent blistering.

Sitz Bath: Use two to three drops only because of potential skin irritation. This is a remarkable aid that helps reduce discomfort in the lower part of the body.

Showers: Add two to three drops of essential oils to your sponge or washcloth and rub over your body during shower.

Dry Brushing: Add two or three drops to your special brush/glove to stimulate your skin and your lymphatic system. All over the body, massage the glove from the toes up to the heart, from the fingers to the heart, always working from the extremities toward the heart. This is very effective before or after your morning shower, once a week.

MARINA MERMAID PRODUCTS

Legend: ⭐ denotes my products
ꕀ denotes products I recommend
✿ denotes blends, handmade, or single essential oils

⭐ Lip Balm

Lick & Bite

✿ Inhalers

Nose Job Crystal Clear
Nose Job Sports
Nose Job I Believe
Nose Job Pure Potential
Nose Job Limitless

✿ Single oils

Bergamot

Bay Laurel

Benzoin

Black Pepper

Camphor

Cardamom

Carrot Seed Oil

Cedar

Cedarwood

Cinnamon

Citronella
Clary Sage
Clove
Coriander
Eucalyptus
Fir
Fennel
Frankincense
Geranium
German Chamomile
Ginger
Grapefruit
Helichrysum
Jasmine
Juniper
Lavender
Lemon
Lemongrass
Lime
Mandarin
Marjoram
Melissa
Myrrh
Neroli
Orange: Sweet/Bitter/Blossom/Blood
Palmarosa
Patchouli

Pine

Peppermint

Petitgrain

Ravensara

Rose

Rosemary

Sage

Sandalwood

Spearmint

Spruce

Tangerine

Tea Tree

Thyme

Ylang Ylang

 Blends

Belly Zen (Anti-Gas)

Breath Booster (Chest Rub)

Buddha Flush (Anti-Cellulite)

Chillax (Chill & Relax)

Detox the Cleaner (Anti-Food Poisoning)

Digestive Warrior (Digestive Aid)

Doggy Styles (Dog Relaxation Aid)

Dragon Lady Flush PMS

Dragon Lady Flush Dysmenorrhea

Dragon Lady Flush Hot Flash

Flow (Constipation)

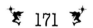

Headache Gooone
Mister Fix it R (Relaxation)
Mister Fix it M (Muscles)
Mister Fix it B (Bones)
Parasites in Me? No way!
Pump the Joy (Uplifter)
Pump the Peace (Anti-Stress)

❀ Perfume Body Oils

Flow (Uplifter)
Sexy Mermaid (Attraction)
Wanted (Aphrodisiac)

❦ Body Lotions

After Sex Glow
Aloha Mermaid
Buddha Yoga Fresh
Creamsicle
Gladiator Awakening
Marie-Jeanne de France

❦ Gel Soaps

After Sex Glow
Buddha Yoga Fresh
Creamsicle
Gladiator Awakening
Lavender de France

❀ Spritzers

Chillax (Chill & Relax)

Dragon Lady Flush PMS

Dragon Lady Flush Dysmenorreah

Dragon Lady Flush Hot Flash

Green Wing (Afternoon Facial Spray)

Pump the Joy (Uplifter)

Pump the Peace (Anti-Stress)

Salute the Sun (Morning Facial Spray)

White Wing (Evening Facial Spray)

❦ MARINA MERMAID First Aid & Travel Kit

(Includes 13 Single oils)

Clove

Eucalyptus

German Chamomile

Geranium

Ginger

Grapefruit

Lavender

Lemon

Lemongrass

Patchouli

Peppermint

Tea Tree

Thyme

✿ Carrier Oils

Jojoba Oil

Apricot Kernel Oil

Almond Oil

✦ Recommended Wellness Accessories

10 ml Sleek Portable 5"x 5/8" Plastic Spritzer Bottles

Renaissance Glove (you can order this through me)

Tab Bra www.tabbra.com

Car Diffuser (you can order this through me)

Mist de Light Ultrasonic Ionizer & Diffuser (you can order this through me)

Spiritual Gangster clothing www.maayoga.com

Amazing Cleansing Programs www.cleansing. marinadufort.com

FOOD "Ash" pH

The following is a list of common foods with an approximate, relative potential of acidity (-) or alkalinity (+), as present in one ounce of food.

Alfalfa Grass	+29.3
Almond	+3.6
Apricot	-9.5
Artichokes	+1.3
Asparagus	+1.1
Avocado (Protein)	+15.6
Banana, Ripe	-10.1
Banana, Unripe	+4.8
Barley Grass	+28.7
Barley Malt Syrup	-9.3
Beans, French Cut	+11.2
Beans, Lima	+12.0
Beans, White	+12.1
Beef	-34.5
Beer	-26.8
Beet Sugar	-15.1
Beet, Fresh Red	+11.3
Biscuit, White	-6.5
Blueberry	-5.3
Borage	+3.2
Brazil Nuts	-0.5
Bread, Rye	-2.5
Bread, White	-10.0
Bread, Whole-Grain	-4.5
Bread, Whole-Meal	-6.5
Brussels Sprouts	-1.5

Buckwheat Groats	+0.5
Butter	-3.9
Buttermilk	+1.3
Cabbage, Green (December Harvest)	+4.0
Cabbage, Green (March Harvest)	+2.0
Cabbage, Red	+6.3
Cabbage, Savoy	+4.5
Cabbage, White	+3.3
Cantaloupe	-2.5
Caraway	+2.3
Carrot	+9.5
Cashews	-9.3
Cauliflower	+3.1
Cayenne Pepper	+18.8
Celery	+13.3
Cheese, Hard	-18.1
Cherry, Sour	+3.5
Cherry, Sweet	-3.6
Chia, Sprouted	+28.5
Chicken	-18.0 to -22.0
Chives	+8.3
Coconut, Fresh	+0.5
Coffee	-25.1
Comfrey	+1.5
Corn Oil	-6.5
Cranberry	-7.0
Cream	-3.9
Cucumber, fresh	+31.5
Cumin	+1.1
Currant	-8.2
Currant, Black	-6.1
Currant, Red	-2.4

Dandelion	+22.7
Date	-4.7
Dog Grass	+22.6
Eggs	-18.0 to -22.0
Endive, Fresh	+14.5
Fennel	+1.3
Fig Juice Powder	-2.4
Filbert	-2.0
Fish, Fresh Water	-11.8
Fish, Ocean	-20.0
Flaxseed Oil	-1.3
Flaxseed	+3.5
Fructose	-9.5
Garlic	+13.2
Gooseberry, Ripe	-7.7
Grapefruit	-1.7
Grapes, Ripe	-7.6
Hazelnut	-2.0
Honey	-7.6
Horseradish	+6.8
Juice, Natural Fruit	-8.7
Juice, White Sugar Sweetened Fruit	-33.4
Kamut Grass	+27.6
Ketchup	-12.4
Kohlrabi	+5.1
Lecithin, Pure (Soy)	+38.0
Leeks (Bulbs)	+7.2
Lemon, Fresh	+9.9
Lentils	+0.6
Lettuce	+2.2
Lettuce, Fresh Cabbage	+14.1
Lettuce, Lamb's	+4.8

Limes	+8.2
Liquor	-28.6 to -38.7
Liver	-3.0
Macadamia Nuts	-11.7
Mandarin Orange	-11.5
Mango	-8.7
Margarine	-7.5
Marine Lipids	+4.7
Mayonnaise	-12.5
Meats, Organ	-3.0
Milk Sugar	-9.4
Milk, Homogenized	-1.0
Millet	+0.5
Molasses	-14.6
Mustard	-19.2
Nut Soy (Soaked, Then Air Dried)	+26.5
Olive Oil	+1.0
Onion	+3.0
Orange	-9.2
Oysters	-5.0
Papaya	-9.4
Peach	-9.7
Peanuts	-12.8
Pear	-9.9
Peas, Fresh	+5.1
Peas, Ripe	+0.5
Pineapple	-12.6
Pistachios	-16.6
Plum, Italian	-4.9
Plum, Yellow	-4.9
Pork	-38.0
Potatoes, Stored	+2.0

Primrose	+4.1
Pumpkin	-5.6
Quark	-17.3
Radish, Sprouted	+28.4
Radish, Summer Black	+39.4
Radish, White (Spring)	+3.1
Raspberry	-5.1
Red Radish	+16.7
Rhubarb Stalks	+6.3
Rice Syrup, Brown	-8.7
Rice, Brown	-12.5
Rose Hips	-15.5
Rutabaga	+3.1
Sesame Seeds	+0.5
Shave Grass	+21.7
Sorrel	+11.5
Soybeans (Cooked, Then Ground)	+12.8
Soy Flour	+2.5
Soy Sprouts	+29.5
Soybeans, Fresh	+12.0
Spelt	+0.5
Spinach (Other Than March)	+13.1
Spinach, March Harvest	+8.0
Straw Grass	+21.4
Strawberry	-5.4
Sugarcane Juice, Dried (Sucanat)	-9.6
Sugarcane juice, Refined (White)	-17.6
Sunflower Oil	-6.7
Sunflower Seeds	-5.4
Sweeteners, Artificial	-26.5
Tangerine	-8.5
Tea (Black)	-27.1

Tofu	+3.2
Tomato	+13.6
Turbinado	-9.5
Turnip	+8.0
Veal	-35.0
Walnuts	-8.0
Watercress	+7.7
Watermelon	-1.0
Wheat Germ	-11.4
Wheat Grass	+33.8
Wheat	-10.1
Wine	-16.4
Zucchini	+5.7

Reproduced by permission of Dr. Robert O. Young, www.phmiracleliving.com

Reference: Young, Robert O. *Sick and Tired.* Alpine, UT, 1977.

The determination of whether a food is acid or alkaline is not gauged by its pH, but the pH of its residue or metabolism.

Books That Keep Me Inspired

Perfume: The story of a Murderer, Patrick Suskind

Words that Shook the World, Richard Greene

101 Reasons Why You Must Write A Book; How to Make a Six Figure Income by Writing and Publishing Your Own Book, Bob Burnham & Jeff McCallum

Miracle Detox Secrets, Tony O'Donnell, Naturopath

Electromagnetic Pollution, A Hidden Stress to Your System, Dr. Sabina M. DeVita

Les Contes du Cordonnier, Pierre Dufort

The Complete Book of Essential Oils & Aromatherapy, Valerie Ann Worwood

Aromatherapy for the Soul, Valerie Ann Worwood

The Art of Aromatherapy, Robert B. Tisserand

Boutique Thinking in a Big Box World, Joe Marcoux

The Illustrated Encyclopedia of Essential Oils, Julia Lawless

Magickal Mermaids and Water Creatures, D.J. Conway

Why Mars and Venus Collide, John Gray

Alkalize or Die, Dr. Theodore A. Baroody

Aromatherapy Workbook, Marcel Lavabre

The Practice of Aromatherapy, Dr. Jean Valnet

The Cure for All Diseases, Hulda Regehr Clark, Ph.D., N.D.

Heal Your Body A-Z, Louise L. Hay

You Can Heal Your Life, Louise L. Hay

The Healing Code, Alexander Loyd, PhD, ND with Ben Johnson, MD, DO, NMD

Ask and It Is Given, Esther and Jerry Hicks

The Law of Attraction, Esther and Jerry Hicks

Magical Mermaids and Dolphins Oracle Cards, Doreen Virtue Ph.D.

Archangel Michael Oracle Cards, Doreen Virtue Ph.D.

Angel Words, Doreen Virtue and Grant Virtue

The Art of Extreme Self-Care, Cheryl Richardson

Essential Women, Jennifer Jefferies

Essential Men, David Webb

Hydrosols, the Next Aromatherapy, Suzanne Catty

The Alchemist, Paulo Coelho

Phoenix Star, Kiernan Antares

Change One Belief, compiled by Bob Burnham

The New Holistic Herbal, David Hoffman

Women's Bodies, Women's Wisdom, Christiane Northrup M.D.

Aromatherapy, Roberta Wilson

Sick and Tired, Dr. Robert O. Young

Want to maximize your health in a natural way?

Take the next step now!

Free Strategy Session: (Value $125.00)

If you have questions about modalities and products discussed in this book and would like to have an enhanced relationship with the oils that is specific to your needs, I'm offering you a <u>free</u> strategy session.

This session **could be the turning point** for a healthier you… and it's totally FREE!

<u>www.MarinaMermaid.com/strategysession</u>

Please note that not all applications for a strategy session are accepted. Only those we feel we can truly help. Massage and wellness practitioners are welcome to apply.

A votre santé,
Marina Dufort RA.

CPSIA information can be obtained at www.ICGtesting.com
Printed in the USA
LVOW101951110312

272577LV00004B/5/P

9 780984 846214